C L I N I C A L
SKILLBUILDERS™

Rapid
Assessment

Springhouse Corporation
Springhouse, Pennsylvania

STAFF

Executive Director, Editorial
Stanley Loeb

Editorial Director
Matthew Cahill

Clinical Director
Barbara F. McVan, RN

Art Director
John Hubbard

Senior Editor
William J. Kelly

Clinical Project Editor
Judith A. Schilling McCann, RN, BSN

Editors
Barbara Delp, Margaret Eckman, Kevin Law, Elizabeth Mauro

Clinical Editors
Maryann Foley, RN, BSN; Mary C. Gyetvan, RN, BSEd

Copy Editors
Jane V. Cray (supervisor), Nancy Papsin

Designers
Stephanie Peters (associate art director), Matie Patterson (senior designer), Linda Franklin

Illustrators
Jean Gardner, Frank Grobelny, Robert Jackson, Robert Jones, Robert Neumann, Judy Newhouse, Robert Phillips, Wendy Wray

Art Production
Robert Perry (manager), Anna Brindisi, Donald Knauss, Thomas Robbins, Robert Wieder

Typography
David Kosten (director), Diane Paluba (manager), Elizabeth Bergman, Joyce Rossi Biletz, Phyllis Marron, Robin Rantz, Valerie Rosenberger

Manufacturing
Deborah Meiris (manager), T.A. Landis, Jennifer Suter

Production Coordination
Colleen Hayman

Editorial Assistants
Maree DeRosa, Beverly Lane, Mary Madden

CS5-010491

Library of Congress Cataloging-in-Publication Data

Rapid assessment.
   p.   cm. – (Clinical Skillbuilders™)
   Includes bibliographical references and index.
   1. Nursing assessment – Handbooks, manuals, etc.   I. Springhouse Corporation.   II. Series.
   [DNLM: 1. Nursing Assessment – handbooks. WY 39 R218]
RT48.R36   1991
610.73 – dc20
DNLM/DLC   90-10450
ISBN 0-87434-364-X

CONTENTS

ADVISORY BOARD AND CONTRIBUTORS

At the time of publication, the advisors held the following positions.

Sandra G. Crandall, RN,C, MSN, CRNP
Director
Center for Nursing Excellence
Newtown, Pa.

Ellen Eggland, RN, MN
Vice President
Healthcare Personnel, Inc.
Naples, Fla.

Terry Matthew Foster, RN, BSN, CCRN, CEN
Clinical Director, Nursing Administration
Mercy Hospital – Anderson
Cincinnati
Staff Nurse, Emergency Department
St. Elizabeth Medical Center
Covington, Ky.

Sandra K. Goodnough-Hanneman, RN, PhD
Critical Care Nursing Consultant
Houston

Doris A. Millam, RN, MS, CRNI
I.V. Therapy Clinician
Holy Family Hospital
Des Plaines, Ill.

Deborah Panozzo Nelson, RN, MS, CCRN
Cardiovascular Clinical Specialist
Visiting Assistant Professor
EMS Nursing Education
Purdue University, Calumet Campus
Hammond, Ind.

Sally S. Russell, RN, MN, CS
Instructor and Clinical Specialist
St. Elizabeth Hospital Medical Center
Lafayette, Ind.

Marilyn Sawyer Sommers, RN, MA, CCRN
Nurse Consultant
Instructor
College of Nursing and Health
University of Cincinnati

At the time of publication, the contributors held the following positions.

Patricia L. Clutter, RN, MEd, CEN
Assistant Nursing Director
Emergency Trauma Center
St. John's Regional Health Center
Springfield, Mo.

Sandra G. Crandall, RN,C, MSN, CRNP
Director
Center for Nursing Excellence
Newtown, Pa.

Pamela J. Currie, RN, MSN, CRNP
Nurse Practitioner
University of Pennsylvania
Philadelphia

Maryann Foley, RN, BSN
Independent Nurse Consultant
Flourtown, Pa.

Mary C. Gyetvan, RN, BSEd
Independent Nurse Consultant
Levittown, Pa.

Cindy S. Hanssen, RN
Emergency Medical Services
Program Coordinator
University of Nebraska Medical Center
Omaha

Kathleen A. Hill-O'Neill, RN, MSN, CRNP
Gerontological Nurse Practitioner
Director of Resident Care
Meadowood Life Care Community
Worcester, Pa.

Sandra Smith Huddleston, RN, MSN, CCRN
Assistant Professor of Nursing
Berea College
Berea, Ky.

Marla Sutton, RN, MSN, CEN
Clinical Nurse Specialist
Emergency Department
Thomas Jefferson University Hospital
Philadelphia

Barbara A. Todd, RN,C, MSN, CRNP
Director, Clinical Services
Cardiac and Thoracic Surgery
Temple University Hospital
Philadelphia

OREWORD

"My chest hurts." "I can't breathe." "My stomach's killing me."

When you hear patient complaints like these, you need to perform a systematic assessment that gives you the pertinent data—fast. But how do you know which questions to ask and what to assess so you get the most information in the least amount of time?

Let's face it. Comprehensive assessment textbooks aren't much help. They tell you how to perform a complete patient assessment—body system by body system. But they don't tell you how to perform a quick assessment of a particular complaint.

For that, you need *Rapid Assessment,* the latest volume in the Clinical Skillbuilders series. Filled with practical information, this book will help you quickly zero in on your patient's chief complaint and analyze your findings.

Rapid Assessment tells you how to assess adult patients with a wide variety of chief complaints. Where appropriate, you'll also find special techniques and considerations for assessing both pediatric and elderly patients.

The book's first three chapters apply to all rapid assessments, regardless of the patient's chief complaint. Chapter 1 gives you an overview of the components of a rapid assessment: the ABCs (airway, breathing, and circulation), general observations, vital signs, history, and physical examination. The chapter goes on to cover the standard physical assessment techniques of inspection, palpation, percussion, and auscultation.

In chapter 2, you'll review how to

check the ABCs and how to open an airway, reestablish breathing, and restore circulation, as necessary. Chapter 3 spells out how and when to make general observations and check your patient's vital signs. In this chapter, you'll also read about how to take a quick, focused history of a patient's chief complaint.

The next four chapters explain how to analyze common chief complaints in each region of the body. Chapter 4 covers the head and neck, including the eyes, ears, nose, and mouth. Chapter 5 focuses on the main organs of the chest—the heart and lungs. Chapter 6 discusses the abdomen, and chapter 7 covers the extremities. Within each chapter, you'll find appropriate history questions for each chief complaint. For example, in chapter 5, you'll see short lists of critical questions for such chief complaints as dyspnea, chest pain, cough, and hemoptysis. Chapters 4 through 7 also explain how and when to use physical assessment techniques for each body region. Plus, these chapters help you interpret your history and physical assessment findings.

Throughout the book, you'll see special graphic devices, known as logos, that alert you to key information. In chapters 4 through 7, the *Anatomy* logo identifies an anatomic illustration of each body region, and the *Checklist* logo accompanies a list of normal findings for each region. You'll also see the *Checklist* logo on other key lists throughout the book; in chapter 1, for example, it accompanies a list of general guidelines for rapid assessment.

Whenever you see the *Diagnostic impression* logo, you'll find a chart that helps you interpret your rapid assessment findings and develop nursing diagnoses. The *Assessment tip* logo signals helpful tips designed to save time or ensure accurate findings. For example, in chapter 1, this logo accompanies a short sidebar on using the stethoscope effectively.

After chapter 7 comes a multiple-choice self-test on rapid assessment. As you'll see, the correct answers follow the last question. After you've read the book, you can use this test to evaluate and further sharpen your rapid assessment skills.

Whether you're a nursing student, a new nurse, or a veteran practitioner, you'll find *Rapid Assessment* indispensable. Unlike any other assessment book, it tells you how to quickly and systematically analyze common chief complaints, using clear language and easy-to-follow illustrations. I urge you to study this book, so you can rapidly assess any chief complaint with ease and confidence.

Mary Snyder Knapp, RN, MSN, CRNP
Vice President
John Whitman & Associates, Inc
Philadelphia

1

FUNDAMENTALS OF RAPID ASSESSMENT

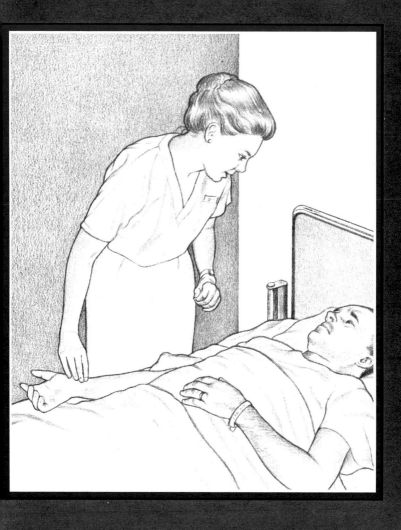

Rapid assessment isn't new. Nurses in critical care units and emergency departments have always performed rapid assessments of their patients.

But today, you need rapid assessment skills no matter where you work. That's because the typical hospital patient is now more acutely ill than ever, and most nurses are busier than ever.

So when you or your patient first notices a change in his condition, you need pertinent information in a hurry. To obtain it, you must have a method for assessing him not only quickly but also systematically. And that's just what this book gives you — a rapid systematic approach to exploring various chief complaints.

In this first chapter, you'll find an overview of the rapid assessment method that's described in detail throughout the book. The chapter also explains how to perform the four assessment techniques — inspection, palpation, percussion, and auscultation. Finally, the chapter describes how to document your rapid assessment.

Components of rapid assessment

Typically, you'll use rapid assessment when a hospitalized patient complains of a change in his condition or when you or someone close to him notices a change in his physical, mental, or emotional status. You may also perform a rapid assessment to confirm a diagnostic finding. For example, if your patient's arterial blood gas analysis indicates a low oxygen content, you'd quickly assess him for other signs of oxygen deprivation, such as an increased respiratory rate and cyanosis.

Rapid assessment includes these components:
- a check of the patient's airway, breathing, and circulation
- general observations
- vital signs
- patient history
- physical assessment.

Keep in mind that you can cover some of these components simultaneously. For example, you can make your general observations of the patient while checking his vital signs or while asking history questions. Remember, your entire assessment shouldn't take very long — probably only a few minutes.

Also remember to be flexible. You won't necessarily use the same sequence for every rapid assessment. The patient's chief complaint and your initial observations will guide your assessment. In some instances, you may not be able to obtain a quick history and instead have to rely on your observations and the information on the patient's chart. (For more information, see *Rapid assessment guidelines.*)

Airway, breathing, circulation
Your first priority will always be to check the patient's ABCs — airway, breathing, and circulation. In many cases, this will consist of just a momentary observation when you first see the patient. But when a patient appears to be unconscious or has difficulty breathing, you'll have to assess his ABCs more thoroughly. If you detect a problem, you'll intervene immediately to reopen the airway, restore breathing, or restart circulation.

General observations
Your general observations may take no longer than 5 seconds. During

this time, you should note the patient's mental status, general appearance, and level of consciousness. These observations should give you clues as to the nature and the severity of his condition.

Remember, learning to make quick, accurate general observations takes time and experience. But such observations will guide you in the proper direction.

Vital signs

The patient's vital signs include his body temperature, pulse, respirations, and blood pressure. Together they give you a quick overview of his physiologic condition, including valuable information on the heart, lungs, and blood vessels.

The seriousness of a patient's chief complaint as well as your general observations of his condition will determine how extensively you measure vital signs. If, for example, a patient has chest pain and shortness of breath, you may have time for only a cursory count of his respiratory rate before you must intervene.

A patient's age, activity level, and physical and emotional condition may affect his vital signs. So always compare a patient's vital signs with his baseline values. You can also use vital signs to monitor a patient's response to interventions and to determine the need for further intervention.

Patient history

During the patient history, you'll learn about the patient's perception of his chief complaint. Use the history to clarify, expand on, and organize information about the chief complaint.

Sometimes what appears to be the chief complaint is actually a secondary problem. So explore the pa-

CHECKLIST

Rapid assessment guidelines

When you perform a rapid assessment, these guidelines will help you focus on the problem, ensure a thorough evaluation, and keep the patient calm.

□ *Identify yourself.* If you don't know the patient, introduce yourself by name and title, and tell him you can help. Given the wide variety of uniforms worn in hospitals today, a patient and his family may not know you're a nurse unless you identify yourself. This becomes especially important in an emergency—a time when the patient must know he's getting the help he needs. If a patient is unconscious, quickly identify yourself to family members or other visitors.

□ *Stay calm.* A calm, orderly approach will help you gain the patient's confidence. And if your demeanor can reduce his anxiety, you're more likely to get accurate information from him.

□ *Avoid tunnel vision.* When performing a rapid assessment, you sometimes must look past a striking problem to see a life-threatening one. For example, you can become so preoccupied with an accident victim's fractured bone that you don't notice pupillary changes that may indicate a serious head injury.

□ *Avoid quick conclusions.* Similarly, you need to maintain a systematic approach and guard against drawing conclusions too quickly. In particular, you shouldn't assume that the patient's current complaint is related to his admitting diagnosis. Use your patient history and physical examination to collect appropriate information. Then draw your conclusions.

tient's complaint with pointed questions. Find out what's bothering him the most. Then get him to quantify the problem. Does he, for instance, feel worse today than he did yesterday? Such questions will help you focus your assessment.

Of course, you won't always be interviewing the patient himself. If he can't respond, you may have to obtain pertinent information from a family member or friend. You can also consult the patient's chart.

Physical assessment

To perform the physical assessment, you need to work rapidly, systematically, and efficiently. This saves you time and helps you establish your priorities.

Begin by concentrating on the areas related to the patient's chief complaint. For example, if the patient complains of abdominal pain, focus the physical examination on his abdomen. Compare the results of this examination with baseline data, if possible.

In some special cases, you may have to perform a complete head-to-toe or body systems assessment — for instance, if a patient is unresponsive (yet has no breathing or circulatory problems) or if a patient is confused and thus unreliable. But in most cases, your physical assessment will be guided by the chief complaint as well as by your general observations and vital signs findings.

Physical assessment techniques

When performing the physical assessment, you'll use a combination of tools and techniques. The tools you'll use include four of your senses — touch, sight, hearing, and smell — along with instruments that

enhance your senses such as a stethoscope, sphygmomanometer, and penlight. The techniques you'll use are inspection, palpation, percussion, and auscultation.

Inspection

The most frequently used assessment technique, inspection can reveal more than the other techniques — when it's performed correctly. Unlike palpation, percussion, and auscultation, inspection isn't a single self-contained assessment step. Instead, it begins when you first see the patient and continues as you check ABCs, make general observations, measure vital signs, take a history, and perform a physical assessment.

Inspection should give you an overall picture of a patient's health and point out any striking characteristics. With a thorough and accurate inspection, you'll notice changes in your patient that indicate improvement or deterioration in his condition, or the presence of a new problem.

Inspection techniques. To ensure a complete inspection, develop a systematic method you can use routinely. (Occasionally, you may have to adjust your method to accommodate individual patients.)

One method is to mentally divide the patient's body into sections. Then zero in on each section, using the same sequence every time. Moving along the body in this manner helps you spot any obvious physical problems. If a complete head-to-toe assessment is necessary, inspect the patient by starting at the forehead and working your way down the body.

When you focus on the area related to the patient's chief complaint, note any landmarks and the

Improving your palpation technique

You can improve your palpation technique by taking advantage of the tactile sensitivities specific to each region of the hand.

The *tips and pads of the fingers* can best distinguish texture and shape and detect lymph node enlargement.

The *ball of the hand* (at the base of the fingers on the ventral surface) can best detect thrills (fine vibrations over the precordium), fremitus (tremulous vibrations over the chest wall), and vocal vibrations through the chest wall.

The *thumb and index finger* can best assess hair texture and grasp tissues.

The *flattened finger pads* can best palpate tender tissues, feel for crepitus (crackling) at the joints, and lightly probe the abdomen.

The *back of the hand, or dorsal surface*, can best detect temperature changes.

The *whole hand* can best test handgrip strength.

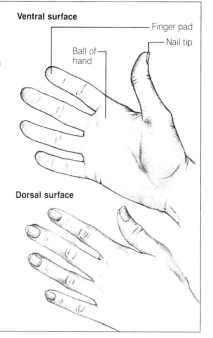

Ventral surface

Finger pad

Nail tip

Ball of hand

Dorsal surface

area's overall condition. Quickly inspect the area's size, shape, texture, position, and color and note any movement. If appropriate, compare body structures for symmetry with contralateral structures.

Nursing considerations. Make sure you perform your inspection in a well-lit room. Either good overhead lighting or sunlight is essential for an accurate inspection. Note the room's temperature; heat and cold can affect skin color.

As you inspect, your initial impressions from the patient history will be strengthened or weakened. Guard against looking only for predictable physical findings. Precon-

ceived ideas of what you should find may distort your actual findings.

Palpation

Usually, you'll palpate immediately after inspection. Sometimes though, this sequence will be altered — for instance, during an abdominal assessment, you won't palpate until after you've auscultated and percussed to avoid affecting bowel sounds and percussion sounds.

The skilled use of touch, palpation helps you obtain further clinical information. With your fingers and hands you can determine the size, shape, and position of many body structures, as well as assess their texture and movements. You can

Performing palpation techniques

To perform rapid assessment, you'll need to master the palpation techniques described below.

Light palpation of a pulse

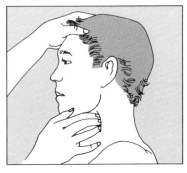

Using the lightest touch possible, press the skin about ½″ to ¾″ (1 to 2 cm).

Light palpation of abdomen

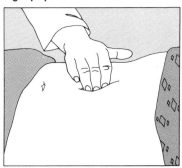

Hold your hand parallel to the abdomen and your fingers together. Then depress the abdominal wall about ½″ to ¾″, as shown.

palpate such structures as the thyroid gland, lymph nodes, blood vessels, and abdominal organs. (Of course, during a particular rapid assessment you'll limit palpation to the area of the chief complaint.)

Using palpation, you can elicit tenderness, guarding, and rebound tenderness and help identify distention and aortic enlargement in the abdomen. With this technique, you can also check a pulse and detect muscle spasm, vibration (fremitus), rigidity, and crepitus. Plus, you can assess the extent of pain or swelling.

Palpation techniques. The more you perform palpation, the better your technique becomes. To improve your skills, learn the sensitivities of the different parts of your hands and

fingers and use them in your physical assessment (see *Improving your palpation technique,* page 5).

During your assessment, you may use light palpation and deep palpation. You'll use light palpation primarily to detect slight tenderness and assess muscle tone. Keep your hand parallel to the body surface being examined and keep your fingers together. Then gently depress the skin and move your fingers in a circle.

Deep palpation helps you identify abdominal organs and masses. You may use one or both hands. Keep in mind that deep palpation may cause patient discomfort. (See *Performing palpation techniques.*)

Nursing considerations. Remember that touching a patient may create

Deep palpation of abdomen

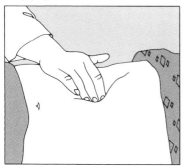

For deep palpation with one hand, extend your fingers as shown. Then depress the abdominal wall about 2″ (4 cm).

Bimanual deep palpation of abdomen

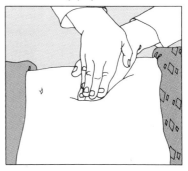

To perform bimanual deep palpation, place the palm of one hand on the abdomen. Then place your other hand on top of the first, as shown. Depress the abdomen evenly to a depth of about 2″.

embarrassment or fear, so always explain what you're doing, why you're doing it, and what discomfort, if any, the patient can expect.

To reduce muscle tension that may interfere with palpation, encourage the patient to relax by having him breathe slowly and deeply through his mouth. Also, avoid palpating tender areas until last.

Finally, watch the patient's facial expressions for signs of pain during your palpation. If you elicit pain, stop palpating.

Percussion

You'll use percussion for two basic purposes: to produce percussion sounds and to elicit tenderness. Percussing for sound, the more common purpose, helps you determine the size, shape, position, and density of underlying organs. It also can help you detect fluid or air in a body cavity.

To percuss for sound, you'll use quick, sharp blows against the patient's body surface (usually the chest or abdomen). These blows create vibrations that penetrate about 1½″ to 2″ (4 to 5 cm) under the skin. The vibrations, in turn, generate distinct sound waves, depending on the density of the underlying structure. The denser the structure, the duller the sound. The five percussion sounds you'll hear are resonance, tympany, dullness, hyperresonance, and flatness (see *Identifying percussion sounds,* page 9).

To accurately compare percussion sounds, use the same force over each area. Note any unexpected sounds — for instance, dullness over

Performing percussion techniques

You should be familiar with the three percussion techniques: indirect, direct, and blunt percussion.

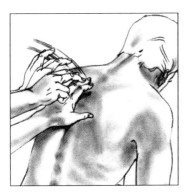

Indirect percussion

To perform indirect percussion, place the distal phalanx of the middle finger on your nondominant hand against the patient's body surface. (This finger that will be struck is known as the pleximeter.) Then, keeping the wrist of your dominant hand loosely flexed, strike the pleximeter with the tip of your dominant middle finger (called the plexor). As you deliver the blow, the plexor should be perpendicular to the pleximeter. Remove the plexor immediately after delivering the blow; otherwise, you'll muffle the sound.

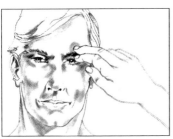

Direct percussion

This technique helps you assess an adult's sinuses for tenderness or elicit sounds in a child's thorax. To perform direct percussion, strike the patient's body surface directly with your hand or fingertip.

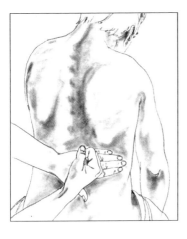

Blunt percussion

Blunt percussion can be performed in two ways. Both elicit tenderness over such organs as the kidneys, gallbladder, or liver; neither is intended to create sounds.

With the first technique you strike the patient's body surface using the ulnar surface of your fist. With the second technique, you place the palm of your nondominant hand over the area to be percussed. Then, strike the back of that hand with the fist of your dominant hand, as shown.

Note: Never perform blunt percussion over the thorax of an elderly patient because the ribs can easily fracture.

Identifying percussion sounds

Percussion sounds vary, depending on the underlying tissue. This chart lists the important percussion sounds, their qualities, and typical locations.

SOUND	QUALITY	LOCATION
Resonance	Hollow	Normal lung
Tympany	Drumlike	Stomach and intestine
Dullness	Thud	Liver; full bladder; enlarged spleen; impregnated uterus
Hyperresonance	Booming	Hyperinflated lung (as in emphysema)
Flatness	Flat	Muscle

an area where you should hear resonance.

Percussion techniques. Depending on the body area you're examining and the purpose of percussion, you'll use one of three methods: indirect, direct, or blunt percussion. The most commonly used method, indirect percussion produces clear, crisp sounds when performed properly. Direct percussion has limited uses — eliciting tenderness in an adult's sinuses and producing percussion sounds in a child's thorax. Blunt percussion is used only to elicit tenderness. (For more information, see *Performing percussion techniques.*)

Use the following tips to enhance your technique and improve your percussion skills:

• Before you start, make sure you have short fingernails and warm hands.

• Ask the patient to void before you begin; otherwise, you may mistake a full bladder for a mass or cause the patient unnecessary discomfort.

• Eliminate as much noise in the room as possible.

• Remove jewelry or other items that may clatter and interfere with your ability to hear percussion sounds.

• When percussing for sounds, organize your percussion sequence so you move from more resonant body areas to less resonant ones. This helps you recognize changes more easily.

• Expect percussion sounds in an obese patient to be muffled by a thick subcutaneous fat layer. You can improve the sound quality by placing the lateral aspect of your thumb on the patient and tapping sharply on the last thumb joint with your other finger.

• Because blunt percussion may startle or upset an unprepared patient, briefly explain to him what you'll be doing and why.

Auscultation

The final part of physical assessment, auscultation involves listening to body sounds — particularly those produced by the lungs, heart, blood vessels, stomach, and intestines. Although you can perform auscultation directly over a body surface using

Components of a dual-head acoustic stethoscope

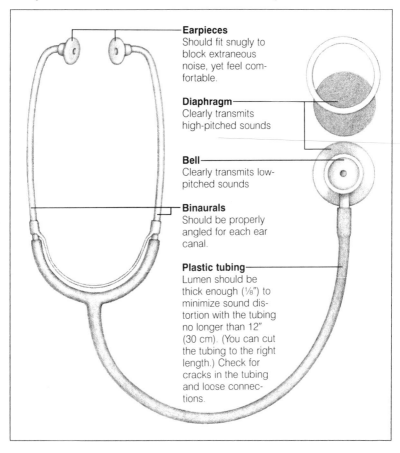

Earpieces
Should fit snugly to block extraneous noise, yet feel comfortable.

Diaphragm
Clearly transmits high-pitched sounds

Bell
Clearly transmits low-pitched sounds

Binaurals
Should be properly angled for each ear canal.

Plastic tubing
Lumen should be thick enough (⅛″) to minimize sound distortion with the tubing no longer than 12″ (30 cm). (You can cut the tubing to the right length.) Check for cracks in the tubing and loose connections.

only your ears, you'll typically perform an indirect auscultation with a stethoscope (see *Components of a dual-head acoustic stethoscope*).

To hear low-pitched sounds with the stethoscope, use the bell; to hear high-pitched sounds, use the diaphragm. This means you'll use the bell to hear extra heart sounds, heart murmurs, blood pressure, and bruits. You'll use the diaphragm to hear breath sounds, normal heart sounds, bowel sounds, and friction rubs. (See *Using the stethoscope effectively*.)

Nursing considerations. Keep in mind that many objects, such as bed linen, jewelry, and the patient's gown interfere with the transmission of sound. Even moving your fingers along the tubing or breathing on it can cause interference.

Remember, an acoustic stethoscope only transmits sounds. It doesn't amplify them. If sounds are so distant that they can't be heard with an acoustic stethoscope, use an electronic stethoscope to amplify them.

Documentation

After you've completed your rapid assessment, you need to document your findings and any care given. Documentation, of course, is the primary way of ensuring continuity of care. Thus, you should identify baseline values and help identify, define, and analyze the patient's problem. You also should help establish priorities for treatment.

Documentation substantiates your care, protecting you legally and providing information for audit committees. Your documentation also identifies the professionals involved in a patient's care, justifies their medical and nursing decisions, and reflects the standard of care provided. The patient's record also shows that you obtained an informed consent from the patient and includes his reactions and comments.

How to document
When documenting your rapid assessment, be accurate, concise, and current. Organize your information so other members of the health care team can easily follow it. And try to document your rapid assessment as soon as you finish, using only accepted abbreviations.

While the format of documentation varies from setting to setting, the content shouldn't. For consistency and thoroughness, follow the documentation standards of the Joint Commission on Accreditation of Healthcare Organizations and your hospital's policy.

Using the stethoscope effectively

When using the diaphragm to assess high-pitched sounds, make sure you position the entire surface firmly on the patient's skin.

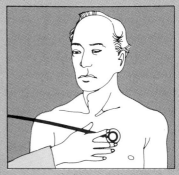

If the patient has hair on his chest, you can reduce extraneous noise and improve contact by applying water or water-soluble lubricant to his chest before auscultating.

When using the bell to assess low-pitched sounds, lightly place the bell on the patient's skin. Exerting pressure can cause the patient's chest to act as a diaphragm and you'll miss low-pitched sounds.

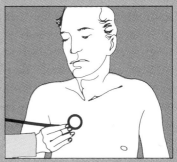

When you have an extremely thin patient, try using a stethoscope with a pediatric chest piece.

What to document

Whenever the patient experiences a sudden change in his condition, be sure to document your immediate general observations, his vital signs, and his history (focusing on the chief complaint). When you ask the patient questions about his chief complaint, write down his exact words using quotation marks.

Always note the source of your information — whether it comes from the patient, a family member, or a friend. If it comes from someone outside the patient's family, state how long the person has known the patient and the nature of their relationship. If you question the reliability of the information, document that as well.

Naturally, you'll document your inspection, palpation, percussion, and auscultation findings. Try to avoid subjective terms such as normal, abnormal, good, or poor. Use specific terms instead. You should also include positive and negative findings.

When you describe the patient's behavior, include only the facts of the behavior — not your opinion on why the patient is behaving a certain way. However, if the patient gives a reason for his behavior, you'll want to document that information.

Finally, be sure to document any intervention taken and the patient's response.

Suggested readings

Fuller, J., and Schaller-Ayers, J. *Health Assessment, A Nursing Approach.* Philadelphia: J.B. Lippincott Co., 1990.

Malasanos, L., et al. *Health Assessment,* 4th ed. St. Louis: C.V. Mosby Co., 1990.

Morton, P.G. *Health Assessment in Nursing.* Springhouse, Pa.: Springhouse Corp., 1990.

2

ASSESSMENT
OF THE
A.B.C.s

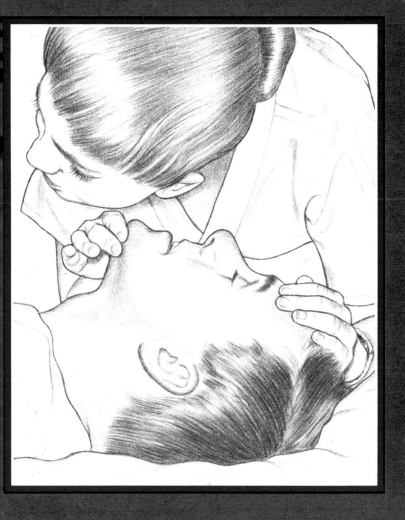

During a rapid assessment, your first priority is to check the patient's vital functions by assessing his airway, breathing, and circulation (ABCs). Many times, you'll perform this assessment in an instant. By the time you first greet the patient and he answers you, you'll have already assessed his ABCs. By answering you, the patient shows that his airway is open, he's able to breathe, and he has a pulse.

But when a patient is unconscious or unable to breathe, you'll have to perform a more detailed assessment. If you detect a problem with his airway, breathing, or circulation, you must intervene immediately — reopening the airway, restoring breathing, or restarting circulation.

This chapter explains how to assess the ABCs of both a conscious and unconscious adult. What's more, you'll find explanations of emergency interventions you may need to perform, including abdominal thrusts and cardiopulmonary resuscitation (CPR).

As you may know, assessing the ABCs of an elderly patient is identical to assessing those of a younger adult. However, you need to be aware of several special considerations when your patient is a child or infant. In the second section of this chapter, you'll find complete explanations of these pediatric considerations.

Assessing adults

Always assess the ABCs in sequence — the airway first, breathing next, and then circulation. As you quickly assess a patient's ABCs, also look for other life-threatening problems that require immediate intervention. If you spot such a problem, take action after your ABC assessment and any necessary interventions.

Assessing the airway
When you assess a patient's airway, note his level of consciousness. Whether he's conscious or unconscious directs, in part, the path your assessment will take and what, if any, interventions you'll perform.

Usually, if a patient has a patent airway, he'll be breathing and have a pulse that indicates adequate circulation. He may or may not be conscious. If a conscious patient doesn't have a patent airway, he'll lose consciousness within a few seconds. At that point, you won't be able to detect breathing, and the pulse will slow and then stop.

Be sure you assess the patient's breathing patterns and level of consciousness quickly and simultaneously. Note whether he seems alert and responsive, difficult to arouse, or nonresponsive.

Conscious patient. To assess a conscious patient's airway, count his respirations and observe his respiratory effort and ability to cough or speak. If a patient appears conscious and able to speak and breathe normally, you can assume that he has a patent airway. If, however, a conscious patient can't cough or speak, or seems to be having trouble breathing, then you should assume he has a completely or partially obstructed airway that requires further assessment. (See *Is your patient's airway obstructed?*)

Listen (without a stethoscope) for breath sounds such as gagging, gurgling, grunting, stridor, snoring, and wheezing — all of which may indicate a partial airway obstruction. Look or asymmetrical chest movements, sternal retractions, diaphoresis, and signs of anxiety — which also may indicate a partial airway obstruction.

If the patient's airway is only partially obstructed, encourage him to cough. This may help clear his airway if, for example, sputum or a mucus plug caused the obstruction. (With elderly patients, dentures are a common cause of airway obstruction.) If the patient can't clear a partial obstruction himself, a complete obstruction will usually develop. If that appears to be happening, ask the patient if he's choking. If his airway is completely obstructed, he won't be able to answer because air can't pass his vocal cords. He may shake his head yes or grab at his throat — a universal distress signal. If this occurs, tell the patient you can help him. Then, with the patient either standing or sitting, perform the abdominal thrust for a conscious patient (see *Positioning for abdominal thrusts,* page 16).

Abdominal thrust. Follow these steps:
• Wrap your arms around the patient's waist and make a fist. Make sure you have a firm grip on the patient because he'll have to be lowered to the floor if he loses consciousness. Check for throw rugs or objects on the floor that may cause you or the patient to slip as you lower him to the floor.
• Place the top of your fist against his abdomen, slightly above the umbilicus and well below the xiphoid process.
• Now grasp your fist with your other hand.
• Press upward and inward with 6 to 10 quick, successive thrusts. The thrusts, which force residual air out

Is your patient's airway obstructed?

When rapidly assessing your patient's airway, suspect a partial or complete airway obstruction if your patient:
☐ develops an increased respiratory rate
☐ begins clutching at his throat
☐ makes crowing noises (stridor)
☐ becomes pale or cyanotic
☐ has exaggerated chest movements, including retractions, especially during inspiration
☐ begins wheezing suddenly or his wheezing increases
☐ develops tachycardia
☐ becomes restless, agitated, fearful, or confused.

Possible causes
Once you identify a blocked airway, you need to look for the cause, which may include:
☐ aspirated food or foreign objects, such as teeth, dentures, or toys
☐ a mucus plug
☐ anaphylaxis
☐ unconsciousness, which causes the tongue to fall back and block the airway
☐ seizures
☐ severe trauma to the face, neck, or upper chest
☐ acute tracheal edema from smoke inhalation or from face and neck burns
☐ allergic reactions to medication.
    You also need to remember that the absence of breathing doesn't always indicate an airway obstruction. The patient may be suffering from something else, such as:
☐ cardiopulmonary arrest
☐ a toxic reaction to an inhaled chemical, an anesthetic, or a drug
☐ respiratory paralysis from a neuromuscular disease, such as myasthenia gravis
☐ a head or spinal cord injury
☐ oxygen toxicity.

Positioning for abdominal thrusts

The illustrations below demonstrate the positions you assume to perform abdominal thrusts on a conscious and an unconscious patient.

With these maneuvers, you use subdiaphragmatic abdominal thrusts to force air from the lungs, thus expelling the foreign body obstructing the airway. To avoid seriously injuring the patient, never place your hands on the xiphoid process or lower rib cage.

Abdominal thrusts on an unconscious patient

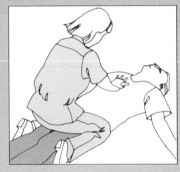

Abdominal thrusts on a conscious patient

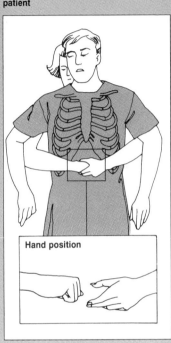

Hand position

of the lungs, should be strong enough to expel a foreign object.

If the patient is pregnant or obese, use chest thrusts instead of abdominal thrusts:
• Stand behind the patient and wrap your arms around his chest. Make sure you have a firm grip.
• Clasp your hands as you did for the abdominal thrusts, but place them in the middle of the sternum with the thumb on your fist inward. Make sure your fist is above the xiphoid process and lower rib cage.
• Quickly and forcefully thrust your fist into the patient's chest, straight back and toward you.

Unconscious patient. If you come upon a patient who appears unconscious, gently shake his shoulders and shout, "Are you okay?" This simple action helps you determine if a patient is unconscious or just sleeping.

If he's unconscious, call for help and place him in a supine position on a hard, flat surface such as the floor. If you suspect a neck injury, logroll him into the supine position to avoid twisting or pulling on his neck, shoulders, and hips.

Next, position yourself near the patient's shoulders. If you don't see signs of breathing, open his airway by repositioning his head using one of two maneuvers. If the patient doesn't appear to have a neck injury, use the head-tilt, chin-lift maneuver. If you suspect a neck injury, use the jaw-thrust maneuver (see *How to open an airway*). In many cases, the muscles controlling the tongue relax, causing the tongue to obstruct the airway, and the maneuver will cause the tongue to fall back in place.

If you see liquid in the patient's mouth, cover your index and middle fingers with a piece of cloth and wipe it out. If you see a solid object, hook it out with your index finger. (You should be aware of the debate surrounding the use of fingers to remove an obstruction. Some health care professionals say you shouldn't try this unless you're sure you can remove the object. They believe the fingers in the mouth create another obstruction.)

Next, place your ear over the patient's nose and mouth and look at his chest to detect air movement, a sign that the airway is clear and the patient has started breathing. If you don't detect breathing, attempt to ventilate him. (See *Guide to ventilation techniques,* page 19.) If that doesn't work, reposition his head and try to ventilate him again. If you still can't ventilate him, perform the abdominal thrust for an unconscious patient. You'll also use this maneuver if a conscious patient with an obstructed airway loses consciousness.

Abdominal thrust. Follow these steps:
● If you haven't already done so, place the patient in a supine position on a hard flat surface.
● Kneel astride his thighs.
● Place the heel of one hand on top of your other hand. Then place your

How to open an airway

If your unconscious patient's tongue blocks his airway, place him on his back and use one of the following two methods to open his airway:

Head-tilt, chin-lift maneuver
Place one hand on the patient's forehead and tilt his head back using firm pressure. Place the fingertips of your other hand under the bony part of the patient's lower jaw, near the chin. Lift the chin, being careful not to completely close his mouth. (Don't place your fingertips on the soft tissue under his chin because this may obstruct the airway you're trying to open.)

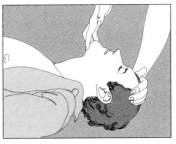

Jaw-thrust maneuver
Position yourself behind the patient's head. Grasp his lower jaw by placing your thumbs on his mandible near the corners of his mouth. Your thumbs should point to his feet and your fingertips should be at the angle of his jaw. Lift his lower jaw with your index fingers while pushing your thumbs down. This causes the patient's jaw to jut forward without hyperextending his neck.

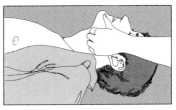

hands between the patient's umbilicus and the tip of his xiphoid process.
• Push inward and upward 6 to 10 times, using enough force to dislodge the object.
• Open the patient's mouth by grasping his tongue and lower jaw with your thumb and fingers. Then lift the jaw.
• If you can see the foreign object, insert the index finger of your other hand deep into the patient's throat at the base of his tongue. With a hooking motion, remove the object.

Now, attempt to ventilate the patient. If this doesn't work, repeat the abdominal thrust and try again to remove the airway obstruction. Continue this pattern until the airway becomes patent or until you begin using advanced life-support measures.

Remember, all of these airway assessments and interventions take place very quickly. Once you know the patient's airway is open, assess his breathing.

Assessing breathing
To assess a patient's breathing, look for his chest to rise and fall, listen for escaped air during exhalation, and feel for a flow of air from the nose and mouth. If you have a stethoscope handy, use it to assess the patient's breathing. Any deviation from the normal respiratory rate of 12 to 16 breaths/minute — or from the patient's baseline respiratory rate — indicates the need for further evaluation.

Conscious patient. Focus your assessment of a conscious patient's breathing on the rate, depth, and character of his respirations. Rapidly assess his skin color and mental status and check for signs of respiratory distress such as a significant

change in respiratory rate and character, dyspnea, retractions, chest pain, and audible breath sounds — including wheezing and gurgling.

If you note any abnormalities, perform a rapid assessment of the lungs and administer oxygen if appropriate. Be sure to notify the doctor of the change in the patient's condition and carry out any new orders. Continue to monitor the patient's respiratory status.

Unconscious patient. Your assessment of an unconscious patient's breathing should take 3 to 5 seconds. First, place him in a supine position, keeping his airway open. Then, place your ear over his nose and mouth. Watch for his chest to rise and fall, listen for the sound of air moving, and feel for the flow of air on your cheek.

If the patient starts to breathe, maintain his airway and continue to assess his breathing until help arrives or until he becomes alert and responsive.

If your assessment reveals no chest movement or air exhalation, begin artificial respirations (also known as rescue breathing), using the following steps:
• With your hand on the patient's forehead, pinch his nostrils closed. If you're using the jaw-thrust method, seal the patient's nostrils by pressing your cheek against them.
• Take a deep breath and then make a tight seal by placing your mouth around his mouth. Depending on the circumstances, mouth-to-mouth ventilations may not be possible (for instance, you may have to give mouth-to-nose ventilations if the patient's mouth is badly injured). If the patient has a stoma, you'll give mouth-to-stoma ventilations. To pro-

(*Text continues on page 22.*)

Guide to ventilation techniques

When your patient requires rescue breathing, you may deliver air from your mouth to his mouth or stoma. To protect yourself from contact with the patient's body fluids, you may use a one-way valve mask.

Mouth-to-mouth

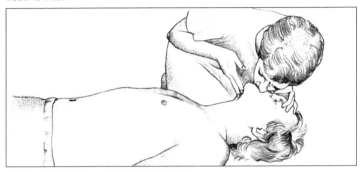

Mouth-to-stoma

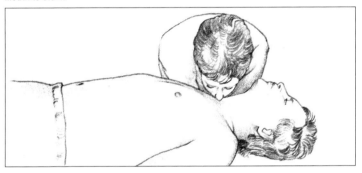

Mouth-to-mask

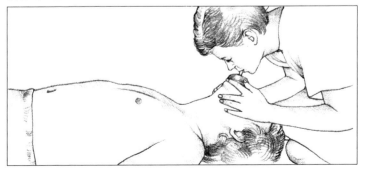

ABCs: When to intervene

The chart below outlines the steps you'll take once you determine that your patient is in distress. (The chart reflects current American Heart Association recommendations.)

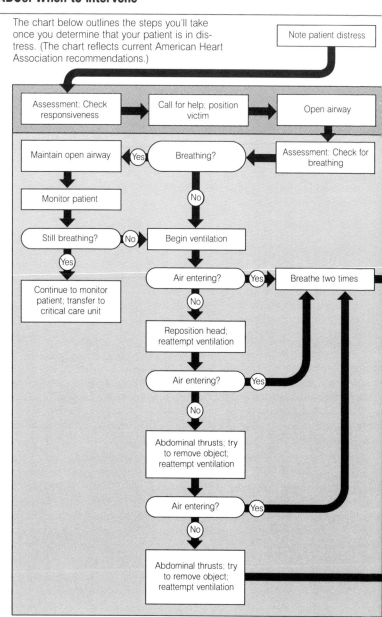

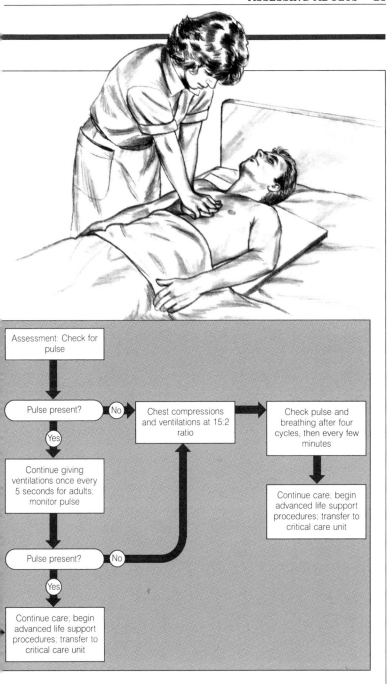

Assessment: Check for pulse

↓

Pulse present? — No → Chest compressions and ventilations at 15:2 ratio → Check pulse and breathing after four cycles, then every few minutes

(Yes)

↓

Continue giving ventilations once every 5 seconds for adults; monitor pulse

↓

Continue care; begin advanced life support procedures; transfer to critical care unit

↓

Pulse present? — No

(Yes)

↓

Continue care; begin advanced life support procedures; transfer to critical care unit tect yourself from the patient's body fluids, you may also deliver mouth-to-mask ventilations. (Keep in mind that you'll need another rescuer if you're using a mask and the patient needs chest compressions; you'll need your hands to hold the mask in place.)

• Give two full ventilations, taking a deep breath after each one. This allows time for the patient's chest to expand and relax and prevents gastric distention. Each ventilation should last 1 to 1½ seconds.

• You can confirm that the air enters and leaves the patient's lungs by watching his chest rise and fall with each breath. You can also listen and feel for air escaping during exhalation. If you don't see the patient's chest move, recheck his head position. Then, making sure you've created a tight mouth seal, try to ventilate him again. If you're still unsuccessful, assume that you're working with an obstructed airway and perform the abdominal thrust for an unconscious patient.

Once you've established the patient's breathing, you can begin assessing his circulation.

Assessing circulation

To check a patient's circulation, you have to assess the function of his heart and vascular network. Do this by checking his skin color, temperature, mental status and, most importantly, his pulse. *Note:* While a pulse tells you blood is moving through the body, it doesn't indicate the rate or degree of perfusion in the body organs.

Use the carotid artery to check a patient's circulation. In a patient with a history of compromised circulation or one who's experiencing a circulatory problem, the radial pulse may not be palpable.

A patient with a palpable pulse may or may not be conscious. However, a pulseless patient will always be unconscious.

Conscious patient. When assessing the circulation of a conscious patient, focus on the rate, rhythm, and character of his pulse. Then auscultate the apical pulse, heart sounds, and blood pressure. During this time, observe the patient's skin color and temperature, as well as his mental status, looking for indications of compromised circulation. A patient whose circulation isn't compromised will usually appear awake and alert with warm, dry, pink skin. Any deviations from this suggest the need for further evaluation.

Unconscious patient. If you find the patient unconscious, place him in the supine position on a hard flat surface, as described above. After assessing his airway and breathing, check his carotid pulse. Keeping one hand on his forehead to keep his mouth open and help maintain airway patency, palpate the carotid artery closer to you with your other hand. (To locate the carotid artery, place your index and middle fingers in the groove between the trachea and the sternocleidomastoid muscle.) Palpate the pulse for about 5 to 10 seconds.

If you detect a pulse, continue to maintain the patient's airway and support his breathing as necessary.

If you can't detect a pulse, the patient needs CPR. (See *ABCs: When to intervene,* pages 20 and 21.)

Performing CPR. First, call for help and then follow these steps:

• Locate the lower margin of the patient's rib cage and move your fingertips along it to the notch where the ribs and the sternum meet.

• Place your middle finger on the

Positioning for two-person CPR

When two rescuers perform cardiopulmonary resuscitation (CPR), the compressor counts out loud with each compression, saying "one and two and three and..." up to five. The ventilator gives a rescue breath at the end of the fifth compression.

After a minimum of 10 cycles, the compressor may call for a switch in positions. Instead of saying "one" she may say, "switch and two and three and four and five." Then the ventilator gives one full breath and moves down to the chest. She finds the landmarks and positions her hands accordingly.

At the same time, the compressor moves to the patient's head, quickly checks for a pulse, and delivers one full breath—initiating a new CPR cycle.

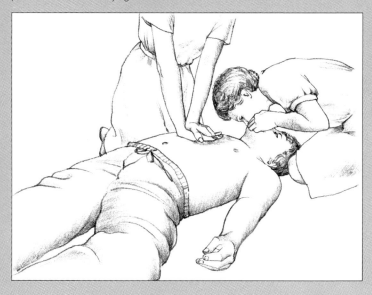

notch and your index finger next to your middle finger so your index finger is on the lower end of the sternum.
● Put the heel of your other hand on the sternum next to your index finger. This aligns the long axis of the heel of your hand with the long axis of the sternum.
● Take your first hand off the notch and put it on top of your hand on the sternum. Make sure you have one hand directly on top of the

other and that your fingers aren't on the patient's chest.
● With your elbows locked, arms straight, and your shoulders directly over your hands, begin chest compressions. Using the weight of your body, compress the patient's sternum 1½″ to 2″ (4 to 5 cm) with the heels of your hands. After each compression, release the pressure and allow the chest to return to its normal position so the heart can fill with blood, but don't remove your

hands from the chest. (Keep in mind that chest compressions may increase the likelihood of fractures in an elderly patient because of osteoporosis.)

Give 15 compressions at a rate of 80 to 100 per minute. Count "one and two and three and..." up to 15, compressing on the number and releasing on "and."

• Remove your hands from the patient's chest and return to his head. Open the patient's airway and administer two ventilations.

• Go back to his chest, reposition your hands using the appropriate landmarks, and deliver 15 more chest compressions and two ventilations. Continue this pattern for four full cycles.

• After completing four cycles, palpate the carotid pulse again. If you don't detect a pulse, continue performing CPR in cycles of 15 compressions and two ventilations, stopping every few minutes to check the carotid pulse.

Continuing CPR. If you're able to detect a pulse, but the patient isn't breathing, give 12 ventilations/minute and monitor his pulse. If at any time, you find you're unable to palpate a pulse, restart chest compressions.

If you're able to detect a pulse and the patient is breathing, continue monitoring his respirations and pulse closely. If his breathing stops, however, resume rescue breathing. If both his breathing and pulse stop, resume CPR.

Stop performing CPR only when the patient's respirations and pulse return, when he's turned over to someone else's care, or when you become exhausted.

If a second person arrives on the scene, let him help you with the CPR. (See *Positioning for two-person CPR,* page 23.) The principles of two-person rescue are the same as above except that you coordinate your efforts with a second person. One person ventilates the patient and checks his pulse, while the other delivers chest compressions. At certain points, the rescuers can switch positions and tasks.

You and the second person compress and ventilate at a ratio of 5:1; that is, you apply five compressions for each one breath.

Assessing infants and children

When assessing ABCs and performing CPR, consider a patient 1 year old or younger to be an infant and consider a patient between ages 1 and 8 to be a child. A patient older than age 8 should be considered an adult.

Basically, you assess the ABCs of an infant or child as you would for an adult, except for the differences explained below.

Assessing the airway

While infants and children have narrower airways than adults, airway assessment remains the same for the three age-groups. The signs of airway obstruction are also the same. And as with adults, the tongue is the most common cause of airway obstruction in infants and children.

The primary respiratory difference between infants and children is that infants are obligate nose breathers. As a result, an infant may experience an airway obstruction because of either nasal secretions or swollen lymph nodes.

Conscious patient. When a conscious infant or child has an obstructed airway, ask his parents if he's recently had a fever or an upper respiratory tract infection while you assess the airway. If he has, you should notify the doctor immediately because the patient may have epiglottitis.

If the patient hasn't had a fever or upper respiratory tract infection, suspect an obstruction caused by a foreign body. You'll perform the abdominal thrust on a child, although if he's small, you'll use less force than you would for an adult. For an infant, you'll use a completely different technique described in the following steps:
• Place the infant face down so he's straddling your forearm with his head lower than his trunk. Support his head by firmly holding his jaw. Rest your forearm and the infant on your thigh.
• With the palm of your hand, deliver four forceful blows to the infant's back between his shoulder blades.
• Put your free hand on the infant's back and support his head. Using both hands, turn him onto your other thigh, making sure his head remains lower than his trunk.
• Place two or three fingers on the sternum, one finger-breadth below the nipple line, and deliver four chest thrusts at a depth of ½" to 1". After each thrust, release the pressure to allow the chest wall to return to the normal position, but don't remove your fingers from the sternum.
• Reassess the patient and continue the pattern of back blows and chest compressions until the patient expels the foreign object or becomes unconscious.

Unconscious patient. If you come upon a pediatric patient who appears unconscious and you suspect an airway obstruction, intervene using these steps:
• Call for help. If the patient's parents are present, ask them what happened while you place the patient in a supine position on a hard flat surface.

For a child:
• Follow the same procedure as you would for an unconscious adult who you suspect has an airway obstruction. If you need to perform the abdominal thrust on a small child, remember to use less force.

For an infant:
• Gently shake him to determine his level of consciousness.
• If you don't get a response and you don't suspect a head or neck injury, use the head-tilt, chin-lift maneuver to open the infant's airway. Be careful not to hyperextend the neck as you tilt the head back; otherwise, the tongue may block the airway. If you suspect a head or neck injury, use the jaw-thrust maneuver to open the airway. Now, attempt to ventilate the patient.
• If neither of these maneuvers opens the infant's airway, administer four back blows and four chest thrusts.
• Now, whether the infant was unconscious when you came upon him or he became unconscious while you were treating him for an obstruction, place your thumb in his mouth on top of his tongue and wrap your fingers around the lower jaw. Then pull the tongue and jaw forward. Look for the object and remove it with your index finger if you see it. Don't try to remove an object unless you can actually see it.
• Continue the airway maneuver, back blows, chest thrusts, and inspection until you remove the object or until you begin advanced life-support measures.

Assessing the brachial pulse

When assessing circulation, you use the carotid pulse in all patients *except* infants. With an infant, you assess the brachial pulse as shown in the illustration below.

While maintaining the head tilt with one hand, palpate the brachial pulse with the other. You'll find the brachial artery on the inside of the upper arm. Use your index and middle fingers to palpate the pulse.

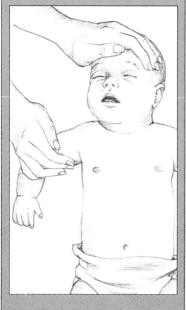

Assessing breathing

Pediatric patients require twice as much oxygen as adults, causing them to breathe faster. Pediatric patients also have limited compensatory mechanisms. Their immature intercostal muscles, weak accessory muscles, and immature rib cartilage make them primarily abdominal breathers.

Despite such differences, your rapid assessment of a child's or infant's breathing will be much the same as it would be with an adult. When assessing a pediatric patient with respiratory difficulty, you'll often find a respiratory rate above baseline, nasal flaring, and sternal retractions.

Conscious patient. With a conscious pediatric patient, you'll focus your breathing assessment on the rate, depth, and character of his respirations. As with an adult, you'll also rapidly assess the patient's skin color and mental status, as well as check for signs of respiratory distress—such as sternal retractions and abnormal breath sounds (respiratory stridor and wheezing). If you note any abnormalities, administer oxygen, notify the doctor, carry out any new orders, and continue to monitor the patient's respiratory status.

Unconscious patient. To assess the breathing of an unconscious pediatric patient, place your ear over his nose and mouth. Look, listen, and feel for air movement. If you detect air moving, continue to maintain his airway and closely monitor his breathing.

If you don't detect air moving, begin rescue breathing as before. With an infant, however, you'll make the following modifications:
• Make a tight seal over the infant's mouth and nose with your mouth.
• Give two ventilations, pausing between them to take a breath yourself. Remember that an infant's air passages are small. So deliver enough breath to make the chest expand, but not so much that you cause gastric distention or barotrauma.
• If you still feel no air movement,

ey differences in CPR techniques

When you perform cardiopulmonary resuscitation (CPR), your technique will depend on the patient's age.

	ADULT (> 8 YEARS)	CHILD (1 TO 8 YEARS)	INFANT (< 1 YEAR)
Ventilations/ minute	12	15	20
Compression delivery	Heels of both hands	Heel of one hand	Middle and ring fingers
Compression depth	1½" to 2"	1" to 1½"	½" to 1"
Compression-ventilation ratio	15:2 (one rescuer) 5:1 (two rescuers)	5:1 (one rescuer) 5:1 (two rescuers)	5:1 (one rescuer)

position the infant's head and try gain. If necessary, take measures o clear an obstructed airway.

ssessing circulation

ou assess the circulation of a child uch as you would that of an adult, sing the carotid artery. However, ith an infant you'll palpate the rachial pulse because the carotid ulse may not be accessible in an ifant's short neck. (See *Assessing e brachial pulse.*)

onscious patient. When assessing e circulation of a conscious infant r child, palpate the appropriate ulse for 5 to 10 seconds. Be sure to ssess the rate, rhythm, and character, noting any abnormalities. Folw up with a rapid cardiac ssessment.

nconscious patient. When assessg the circulation of an unconscious ifant or child, you also should palate the appropriate pulse for 5 to 0 seconds.

If the patient has a pulse but isn't reathing, perform rescue breathing ntil he resumes breathing. With a

child, deliver a breath every 4 seconds — a rate of about 15 breaths/ minute. With an infant, deliver a breath every 3 seconds — a rate of about 20 breaths/minute.

If you don't detect a pulse, perform CPR, making the necessary modifications for an infant or a child (see *Key differences in CPR techniques*).

For a child, make these modifications:
• Compress the chest with the heel of one hand (see *Positioning for pediatric chest compressions,* page 28). With a large child, use two-handed chest compression as you would with an adult.
• Compress the chest at the same rate of 80 to 100 times per minute, but to a depth of 1" to 1½" (2.5 to 3 cm).

For an infant, make these modifications:
• Imagine a line drawn between the nipples. Place the index finger of your free hand on the sternum, just below this line. Then place your middle and ring fingers next to your index finger on the sternum.
• Lift your index finger off the

Positioning for pediatric chest compressions

These illustrations show how to position your fingers or hand to compress the chest of an infant or a child during cardiopulmonary resuscitation. For an infant, measure one fingertip width down from the nipple line and perform compressions with your middle and ring fingers, as shown. For a child, place the heel of your hand two fingertip widths above the point where the ribs meet the sternum, as shown.

Finger position for infant chest compression

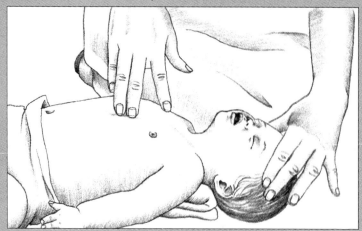

Hand position for child chest compression

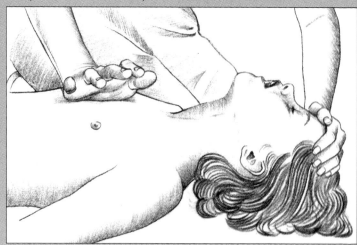

chest. Then, using only your middle and ring fingers, deliver five chest compressions, at a rate of at least 100 per minute. Compress to a depth of ½" to 1" (1 to 2 cm). Release the pressure after each compression, allowing the chest wall to return to its normal position.
• Keeping one hand in the proper position on the infant's chest, use your other hand to maintain the airway with the head-tilt maneuver.
• Give compressions and ventilations at a ratio of 5:1 for a total of 10 cycles.

Recheck the infant's pulse. If you can't detect one, continue with CPR and check the pulse every few minutes.

Suggested readings

Albarran-Sotelo, R., et al. *Textbook of Advanced Cardiac Life Support.* Dallas: American Heart Association, 1987.

Britt, J. "What To Do When Your Patient Codes," *Nursing90* 20(1):42-43, January 1990.

Deshpande, V.M., et al. *Comprehensive Examination Review for Respiratory Care Practitioners.* East Norwalk, Conn.: Appleton & Lange, 1988.

Finucaine, B.T., and Santora, A.H. *Principles of Airway Management.* Philadelphia: F.A. Davis Co., 1988.

Goldsworth, J. "Cardiac Arrest and Life Support" in *The Handbook of Emergency Nursing: A Nursing Process Approach.* Edited by Mowad, L., and Ruhle, D. East Norwalk, Conn.: Appleton & Lange, 1988.

Holmes, J., and Magiera, L. *Maternity Nursing.* New York: Macmillan Publishing Co., 1987.

Kitt, S., and Kaiser, J., eds. *Emergency Nursing: A Physiologic and Clinical Perspective.* Philadelphia: W.B. Saunders Co., 1990.

Matteson, M.A., and McConnell, E.S. *Gerontological Nursing: Concepts and Practice.* Philadelphia: W.B. Saunders Co., 1988.

Sheehy, S.B. *Manual of Emergency Care,* 3rd ed. St. Louis: C.V. Mosby Co., 1990.

3

PRELIMINARY ASSESSMENT

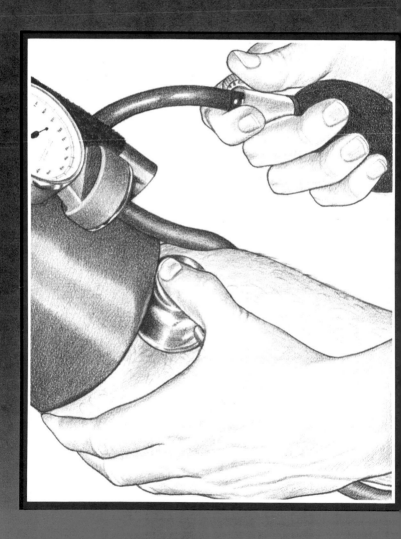

After assessing your patient's airway, breathing, and circulation (ABCs), you're ready to perform a quick preliminary assessment to identify and evaluate his problem. This assessment includes three basic components:

• general observations
• vital signs
  health history.

This chapter gives you the information you need to carry out your preliminary assessment confidently. Keep in mind that your preliminary assessment findings will help guide your subsequent physical assessment of the patient.

General observations

Your broad observations of the patient include noting his mental status, overall appearance, and level of consciousness (LOC). Actually, you'll begin to make general observations—particularly about mental status and overall appearance—when you first meet the patient. After you've assessed (and, if necessary, stabilized) his ABCs, you'll perform a focused assessment of his LOC.

Mental status
When assessing a patient's mental status, pay special attention to his affect. Also evaluate his behavioral and verbal responses for signs of distress, and his speech pattern for abnormal deviations.

Affect. Assess for such signs as hostility, uncooperativeness, restlessness, crying, and poor thought organization. Compare your observations with those reported in previous assessments to detect changes

that may be linked to an underlying disorder.

Even subtle changes in affect may signal impending neurologic or other problems. For instance, a usually cooperative patient who becomes combative may be experiencing intracranial bleeding. A restless patient may be in the initial stage of shock. Don't assume that such a patient is simply uncooperative—you could be overlooking important assessment information.

Behavioral and verbal responses. Assess the patient for signs of distress, such as grimacing, moaning, restlessness, extreme anxiety, and air hunger. Keep in mind that a patient may deny distress. For example, a stoic patient may have a high pain tolerance or refuse to acknowledge pain. Or a patient may believe that denial will ease or vanquish his pain.

Speech pattern. Assess the patient for slurred speech, aphasia, markedly slow or fast speech, and hoarseness. Remember, a deviation doesn't necessarily signal a problem. More significant may be a change from the patient's usual pattern. You can obtain information about his usual pattern from the patient himself, from a family member or other person close to the patient, or from the patient's chart.

Overall appearance
The patient's sex, race, and approximate age will be obvious. Other factors to assess include his skin condition, body type, posture, body movement, obvious deformities, and any unusual odors that may provide a clue to the underlying condition.

Skin condition. Assess the patient's skin for color, noting pallor, cyano-

Recognizing decorticate and decerebrate posturing

Indicating a lesion of the cerebral hemisphere, decorticate (flexor) posturing is marked by unilateral or bilateral elbow, wrist, and finger flexion; shoulder abduction and flexion; internal rotation of the legs; and plantar flexion of the feet.
 Decerebrate (extensor) posturing indicates a lesion in the midbrain or upper

Decorticate posturing

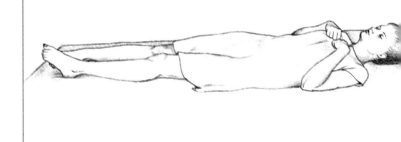

sis, flushing, mottling, or a yellow-orange tint (jaundice). Observe for areas of discoloration (redness, ecchymoses, petechiae, or differences in color between corresponding body areas). Check too for diaphoresis. Assess skin temperature, noting differences between body areas. Also check skin turgor and capillary refill time. (Normal refill time is 2 seconds or less.)

Skin condition can provide important clues to an underlying disorder. For example, pallor and cool, clammy skin can help you identify hypovolemic or cardiogenic shock, and excessive bruising can point to a warfarin (Coumadin) overdose or leukemia.

Body type. Assess the patient's general body type, classifying the build as stocky, average, or slender. Observe for cachexia or obesity. Note any unusual physical features; a barrel chest, for example, may signal chronic lung disease.

Posture. Assessing the patient's posture can provide information on his energy level, psychological status, skeletal structure, and, possibly, neurologic status. Observe particularly for leaning, slumping, hunching forward, and drawing the knees up. Note decorticate (flexor) or decerebrate (extensor) posturing. (See *Recognizing decorticate and decerebrate posturing.*)

Body movement. When possible, observe the patient's gait and other movements for symmetry, coordination, and smoothness. Look for involuntary movements, impaired movement, shuffling, or limping. If your patient is bedridden, focus on his ability to sit up, turn, and reposition himself in bed.

Obvious deformities. Quickly assess for anatomic irregularities, such as fractures and asymmetry of body parts. Evaluate any deformity for clues to an underlying problem.

brain stem. It usually carries a poor prognosis, unless associated with metabolic coma. In this posture, the patient's teeth are clenched; the arms are adducted, extended, and hyperpronated; and the legs are extended with plantar flexion of the feet.

Decerebrate posturing

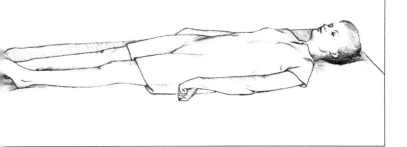

Unusual odors. Note any unusual body odors emanating from the patient, his clothing, or his environment. Certain odors can help you identify problems. For example, halitosis can simply indicate poor oral hygiene but also can point to infection, abscess, cancer, or acute illness. A fecal smell may indicate anaerobic infection, melena, or intestinal obstruction. (See *Detecting distinctive body odors,* page 34.)

Level of consciousness

Quickly determine the patient's LOC by assessing his response to verbal communication, touch, or painful stimuli. Record your findings using an objective scoring system, such as the Glasgow Coma Scale. With this system, you'll be able to detect small changes in the patient's LOC. In some circumstances, you may use the AVPU scale, a way of rapidly characterizing your patient's LOC.

Some clinicians use subjective terms, such as "lethargic," "ob-tunded," and "stuporous" to describe LOC. But this makes it difficult to detect the small changes that can signal important trends.

Glasgow Coma Scale. The most reliable tool for rapidly evaluating LOC, this scale rates the patient's best eye-opening response, best verbal response, and best motor response. (See *Glasgow Coma Scale,* page 35.)

Eye-opening response. First, note whether the patient's eyes open spontaneously. If not, check for an eye opening in response to a verbal stimulus. Speak his name in a normal tone of voice and note his response. If the patient doesn't respond, try gently shaking his shoulder or squeezing his hand.

If neither verbal nor tactile stimulation produces a response, apply a painful stimulus, such as rubbing your knuckles over the patient's sternum or pinching the sternocleidomastoid muscle in the hollow

Detecting distinctive body odors

During your assessment, you may note an odor that provides a clue to an underlying disorder or the ingestion of a toxic or harmful substance. You'll detect certain odors on the breath; others emanate from the body.

ODOR	POSSIBLE CAUSE
• Acetone (on the breath)	Ethanol
• Alcohol (on the breath)	Ethanol, isopropyl alcohol
• Ammonia (on the breath)	Renal failure
• Bitter almond (on the breath)	Cyanide poisoning
• Fecal (from the body)	Anaerobic infection, steatorrhea
• Fecal (on the breath)	Intestinal obstruction
• Fishy (from the body)	Nonspecific vaginitis, ingestion of zinc oxide
• Fruity (on the breath)	Ketoacidosis
• Garlic (from the body)	Arsenic poisoning
• Musty, damp (on the breath)	Pulmonary tuberculosis
• Musty, sweet (on the breath)	Liver failure
• Petroleum distillate, violets (on the breath)	Hydrocarbon poisoning
• Putrid (on the breath)	Lung abscess, bronchiectasis
• Sickly sweet (from the body)	*Pseudomonas* infection

along the top of the shoulder. When applying painful stimuli, be sure you don't cause bruising or other injuries, but apply sufficient pressure to elicit a possible response and avoid reporting a false "no response."

Verbal response. Next, assess the patient's best verbal response. Ask him basic questions— such as "What year is this?"—to determine whether he's fully conscious and responding quickly or whether he's slow to respond.

When assessing the patient's verbal response, be aware of cultural differences, language barriers, and other factors that may influence his ability to respond. Keep your questions clear and simple and be rea-

sonable when evaluating a response When evaluating orientation to place, remember that the patient may be unfamiliar with the area or environment. Also consider that a hospitalized patient—particularly if he's elderly or has recently undergone an involved procedure—may quite naturally lose track of time and dates because he's removed from his normal surroundings and in a stressful environment.

Motor response. Finally, assess the patient's best motor response. Start by asking him to perform simple movements, such as sticking out his tongue or holding up an arm or leg. Don't ask the patient to squeeze your hand. This commonly used technique may elicit a false-positive

Glasgow Coma Scale

The Glasgow Coma Scale provides an easy way to evaluate a patient's level of consciousness and to detect changes from baseline. A decreasing score in one or more categories may signal an impending neurologic crisis.

TEST	REACTION	SCORE
Best eye-opening response	Open spontaneously	4
	Open to verbal command	3
	Open to pain	2
	No response	1
Best verbal response	Oriented and converses	5
	Disoriented and converses	4
	Uses inappropriate words	3
	Makes incomprehensible sounds	2
	No response	1
Best motor response	Obeys verbal command	6
	Localizes painful stimulus	5
	Flexion—withdrawal	4
	Flexion—abnormal (decorticate rigidity)	3
	Extension (decerebrate rigidity)	2
	No response	1
Total		3 to 15

result: You may incorrectly interpret a reflex action as a voluntary movement.

If the patient doesn't obey your verbal command, apply a painful stimulus and record the appropriate score.

After completing your assessment, add the scores from each category to determine a total score indicating LOC. A patient who scores 15 is completely alert, oriented, and able to follow commands. One who scores 7 or less is comatose and probably has severe neurologic damage. A patient with a score of 3 is in a deep coma and has a poor prognosis.

The AVPU scale. When the patient's condition doesn't permit a more thorough examination, you can rapidly characterize his LOC with the AVPU scale:
• A (Alert)
• V (Responsive to verbal stimuli)
• P (Responsive to painful stimuli)
• U (Unconscious).
While useful, this abbreviated assessment tool does not rate or score the patient's level of response as the Glasgow Coma Scale does.

Vital signs

Assessing vital signs — temperature, pulse, respirations, and blood pressure — provides a quick overview of the patient's physiologic status. Vital signs also help you detect important changes in his condition.

When evaluating vital sign measurements, be sure to consider them in relation to your other assessment findings to form an accurate picture of the patient's status. A pulse rate of 45 beats/minute, although of concern, may not be associated with the patient's primary problem. Remember too that vital sign trends usually are more significant than single readings. One borderline hypotensive blood pressure reading may not indicate a shock state.

Compare all findings with the patient's baseline vital signs. An apparently critical reading may be normal for a particular patient. Normal vital signs do vary somewhat among patients, depending on such factors as genetic abnormalities, heredity, underlying physiologic problems, emotional status, medication use, activity level, and even time of day.

Depending on the patient's condition, you may have time for only an abbreviated assessment of vital signs. Initially, you may only estimate blood pressure and quickly count respirations, postponing a more complete assessment until the patient is stabilized. Also, depending on circumstances, you may have to stop your assessment and initiate emergency interventions.

Temperature

Take the patient's oral, rectal, or axillary temperature with a glass or an electronic thermometer. You'll take a rectal or an axillary temperature when the patient is unconscious, confused, disoriented, unable to keep his mouth closed, or receiving oxygen by face mask. If necessary, you can quickly feel the patient's skin for warmth and take his temperature after he's stabilized.

Pulse

The pulse provides information about the cardiovascular system, reflecting the rhythm, rate, and strength of cardiac contractions. A normal pulse rate is between 60 and 100 beats/minute.

Locating a pulse. Begin by quickly locating an appropriate pulse site to palpate. (See *Identifying pulse sites.*) In most adults, you'll find the radial pulse readily accessible and easily palpable. If you can't obtain an accurate radial pulse reading, use an alternate site, such as the carotid, femoral, or apical pulse. The apical pulse provides the most accurate reading but takes the longest to record because you must auscultate instead of palpate.

If you palpate the carotid pulse, avoid exerting excessive pressure, which can stimulate the vagus nerve and cause reflex bradycardia. Also, don't palpate bilateral carotid pulses simultaneously; doing so can impair cerebral circulation.

Assessing pulse rate, strength, and rhythm. First, count the pulse for 15 seconds and multiply by 4 to determine the number of beats per minute. Next, assess the strength and rhythm of the pulse, noting such abnormalities as a bounding pulse; a weak, thready pulse; or an irregular rhythm. If you detect an abnormality, evaluate further with a cardiac monitor.

Identifying pulse sites

This illustration shows the locations of the major peripheral arterial pulses and the apical pulse.

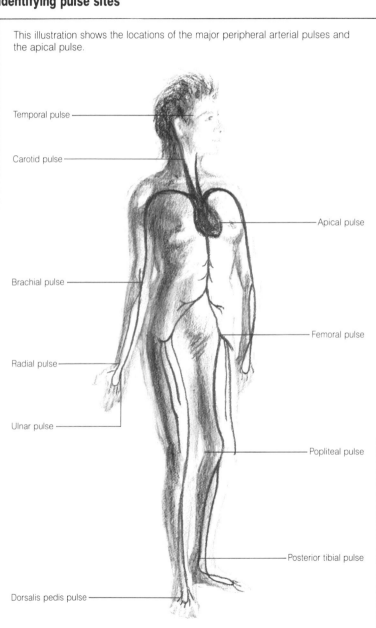

Temporal pulse

Carotid pulse

Apical pulse

Brachial pulse

Femoral pulse

Radial pulse

Ulnar pulse

Popliteal pulse

Posterior tibial pulse

Dorsalis pedis pulse

Generally, a pulse rate above 100 beats/minute indicates tachycardia; a rate below 60 beats/minute, bradycardia. Keep in mind, however, that various factors can cause transient changes in pulse rate. Increases may stem from fear, anger, and pain; decreases, from vomiting, suctioning (causing vagal nerve stimulation), and certain medications. Also, a patient in excellent physical condition may maintain a normal resting pulse rate below 60 beats/minute. As always, consider the entire clinical picture when interpreting your assessment findings.

Respirations

Quickly evaluate the patient's respiratory rate, depth, and rhythm, as well as the ease and regularity of his breathing and chest wall movements. To determine the rate, count all complete respirations for 15 seconds and multiply by 4 to obtain the number of breaths per minute.

To evaluate respiratory depth, observe the rise and fall of the patient's chest and assess the effort he expends to breathe. Describe respirations as shallow, moderate, or deep.

Assess respiratory difficulty by evaluating the patient's breathing pattern or rhythm. Children and adults normally exhibit a regular rhythm, except for occasional sighs. Infants, however, typically exhibit a variable respiratory pattern.

Also observe the patient for use of accessory muscles, such as the scalene, sternocleidomastoid, trapezius, and latissimus dorsi. Using these muscles reflects a weakness of the diaphragm and the external intercostal muscles — the major muscles of respiration. Labored breathing also may cause intercostal muscles to bulge or retract abnormally, as well as nasal flaring and

lip pursing on expiration.

Blood pressure

When you assess your patient's blood pressure, you're measuring the fluctuating force that blood exerts against arterial walls as the heart contracts and relaxes. Arterial blood pressure reflects cardiac output, peripheral vascular resistance, blood volume and viscosity, and arterial elasticity. (See *Factors affecting blood pressure.*) Normal blood pressure ranges from 90/60 mm Hg to 140/90 mm Hg.

Measuring blood pressure. Usually, you'll measure your patient's blood pressure using three pieces of equipment: a sphygmomanometer, an inflatable cuff, and a stethoscope.

The most common site for a blood pressure reading is the arm. When using this site, wrap an appropriate-sized cuff around the upper arm. Then place the diaphragm of the stethoscope over the brachial artery, just below the antecubital area, and auscultate the brachial pulse. (Use the bell of the stethoscope if the patient's pulse is diminished or hard to locate.) When assessing blood pressure in the leg, auscultate over the popliteal artery, keeping in mind that popliteal blood pressure measurements yield higher systolic and lower diastolic readings than those from the brachial artery.

Rapidly inflate the cuff until you can no longer hear the pulse, then continue inflating until the pressure rises another 20 to 30 mm Hg. Slowly open the cuff valve and watch the manometer's mercury column or gauge needle descend. Release the pressure at a rate of about 3 mm Hg/second, and listen for pulse sounds (Korotkoff's sounds). As soon as you hear blood pulsing through the artery, note the reading on the manometer. This is the patient's systolic pressure. Continue deflating the cuff and note the point at which pulsations finally disappear. This is the patient's diastolic pressure.

In a patient with venous congestion or hypertension, you may detect a silent period between the systolic and diastolic sounds when you can't hear intervening pulse sounds. Known as an auscultatory gap, this silence may cause you to underestimate the systolic or overestimate the diastolic reading significantly.

Special considerations. If you can't obtain an audible blood pressure because of severe blood loss, weakened myocardial contractility, or other problems, try to palpate the blood pressure. After applying the cuff, palpate the radial or brachial artery. Inflate the cuff until you can no longer feel the pulse, then deflate slowly. Record the systolic reading as you first feel the pulse again. This procedure lets you palpate only the systolic blood pressure, not the diastolic pressure.

In an emergency, you may have difficulty obtaining a blood pressure reading. If so, you can estimate systolic blood pressure by palpating for pulses at different arterial sites. If you can palpate a carotid pulse, you can assume that the patient's systolic pressure is at least 60 mm Hg; a femoral pulse, at least 70 mm Hg; and a radial pulse, at least 80 mm Hg.

Orthostatic vital signs
To assess orthostatic vital signs, measure pulse rate and blood pressure with the patient supine, sitting, and standing. A pulse rate increase of 10 to 20 beats/minute and a blood pressure decrease of 10 to 20 mm Hg between positions may indi-

Factors affecting blood pressure

Various factors can cause an increase or decrease in blood pressure.

Increased blood pressure may result from:
□ increased cardiac output
□ heightened peripheral vascular resistance
□ expanded blood volume
□ increased blood viscosity
□ diminished arterial elasticity
□ an emotional state (fear, stress, anxiety)
□ pain
□ medications.

Decreased blood pressure may result from:
□ reduced cardiac output
□ decreased peripheral vascular resistance
□ diminished blood volume
□ decreased blood viscosity
□ increased arterial elasticity
□ orthostatic changes
□ medications.

cate hypovolemia, dehydration, or the adverse effects of certain medications.

When performing this simple assessment, be aware that the patient may experience dizziness and even syncope when rising suddenly to a standing position. Prepare him for these possibilities, and be ready to help if they occur.

Health history

The health history provides insight into the patient's perception of his problem. It also helps guide your physical assessment and any emergency interventions.

During a rapid assessment, you'll explore the patient's chief complaint and any pertinent medical history. Even if you have time for only a few questions, the patient's answers can provide important clues to his condition.

You won't always be able to obtain health history data directly from the patient. If he can't respond to your questions, a family member or other person close to the patient may provide essential information. You may also obtain information from the patient's chart. But remember that his current complaint may not be related to his chief complaint on admission or his diagnosis.

Interviewing the patient
To obtain accurate health history information and form a clear picture of the patient's problem, make him feel as comfortable as possible. Actively listen to him. Although you must be careful to differentiate a patient's nervous anxiety from true feelings of impending doom, always take his comments into consideration. When a patient says "I think I'm having an insulin reaction" or "I think I'm going to die," you should immediately explore the problem in more depth.

Whenever possible, ask openended questions to let the patient explain the problem in his own words. Questions requiring yes-orno answers may affect the patient's word choice and discourage him from elaborating. For example, don't ask "Does your pain feel dull?" Instead, ask "What does your pain feel like?"

During the interview, sound reassuring. Any sign of panic on your part may make the patient feel threatened. Also avoid making assumptions; if you act as if you already know what his problem is, he may feel defensive and become discouraged from continuing.

Help a confused or noncommittal patient to clarify his feelings by gradually asking more directed questions. Use as much tact as possible, but be aware that you may have to ask abrupt or potentially embarrassing questions.

Exploring the chief complaint
Evaluating the patient's chief complaint requires adept questioning, knowledge, and experience. As you question the patient, consider that things are not always what they seem. A fairly simple, obvious injury can result from an unexpected underlying cause. For example, careful questioning may reveal that a patient with a simple fracture of the hip fell because of syncope associated with a myocardial infarction, orthostatic hypotension, or the effects of medication.

Begin by eliciting a description of the chief complaint from onset to the present. Start with a general open-ended question to help the patient recall the sequence of events. For example, you might say "Tell me about your problem, from when it first began until now."

Continue by asking more directed questions to elicit more detailed information about the chief complaint and associated symptoms. You can remember important points to cover by using the PQRST device (see *Using the PQRST memory device*).

Exploring medical history
After assessing your patient's chief complaint, quickly review his pertinent medical history. Do so by checking his chart and, if necessary, questioning him (or a family member or another person close to him).

You'll need to cover these important points:

- allergies, including a description of the reaction
- any illnesses requiring treatment
- major surgeries performed (including why and when)
- current medications (both prescription and over-the-counter) and their purposes.

This information allows you to establish a baseline and helps you determine the cause and urgency of your patient's problem. Later, when the patient's condition is stable, you can fill in the other components of a complete health history, including childhood or infectious diseases, prior hospitalizations, immunization history, family history, psychosocial history, and a review of body systems.

Using the PQRST memory device

Use this memory device to make sure you fully explore the patient's chief complaint.

☐ **P**rovoking or palliative factors. What causes the problem? What makes it better? What makes it worse?
☐ **Q**uality or quantity. What does it feel like? Look like? Sound like? How much of it is there?
☐ **R**egion or radiation. Where is it located? Does it spread to other areas?
☐ **S**everity. How severe is it, on a scale of 1 to 10? Does it interfere with normal activities?
☐ **T**iming. When did it begin? Was onset sudden or gradual? How many times has it occurred, and how often?

Pediatric and elderly patients

When you perform a preliminary assessment on a child or an elderly patient, you'll need to modify your approach. The following sections cover the key differences you should be aware of when assessing these patients.

Assessing pediatric patients

You may find rapid assessment a particular challenge with an infant or a child. Consider communication difficulties, for example. A child who hasn't yet mastered language skills can't describe his problem in detail, if at all. So you must be alert for behavior that points to a problem, such as crying, irritability, restlessness, and lethargy. Then, let the child's behavior help guide your assessment. If the child is lethargic, for instance, you'll need to assess LOC.

As when assessing any patient, communicate control and friendliness. Be gentle and considerate, and be positive and direct in all communications. Identify yourself clearly and speak in terms that the child can understand. Above all, be honest when describing procedures; failure to prepare the child for a potentially frightening or painful procedure may destroy his sense of trust in you and other health care providers, interfering with your ability to perform assessments and provide care.

If at all possible, don't separate the child from his parents during your assessment. A child's normal separation anxiety will be heightened in an acute situation. Allowing a parent to stay with the child may help ease anxiety and increase cooperativeness.

General observations. You'll make your general observations in basically the same way you would with an adult. Focus on LOC, affect, behavioral and verbal responses, skin condition, posture, activity level, motor coordination, language, maturity level, and ability to understand and cooperate with the assessment.

Consider that a child may be more spontaneous and restless than an adult. He may stare, ask questions with unabashed curiosity, and readily express emotion.

Observe the patient for signs of anxiety, including thumb-sucking, nail-biting, and rocking. If a parent is present, observe the parent-child interaction.

Note the child's mental status. A sick infant may be extremely irritable or listless, whereas a toddler may sulk or scream. An older child who's sick may be tearful, withdrawn, or irritable. Ask your patient's parents how the child's behavior differs from normal. Unusual behavior tells you something is wrong.

Vital signs. The normal ranges for vital signs vary with age. In general, the younger the child, the lower the blood pressure and the higher the pulse and respiratory rates. (See *Normal pediatric vital signs.*)

Temperature. This measurement is more labile in infants and young children than in older children and adults. For example, a young child's normal rectal temperature may rise as high as 101° F (38.3° C) in the late afternoon. An infant with a severe infection may have a normal or even subnormal temperature, and a young child may have a very high temperature from even a minor infection. So the degree of fever doesn't always correlate with the severity of the illness.

When assessing a child with a febrile illness, keep in mind that you may detect a 10% increase in pulse and respiratory rates for each degree centigrade of temperature increase.

Pulse. You can feel a carotid pulse in an older child, but you may not be able to find it in an infant because his neck is too short. So auscultate his apical pulse, or palpate his brachial pulse.

Note any increase, decrease, or irregularity, remembering that heart rate in infants and children is labile and more sensitive to stressful events. A bounding pulse may indicate a large left-to-right shunt produced by a patent ductus arteriosus. A weak, thready pulse may indicate diminished cardiac output or the presence of peripheral vasoconstriction.

Children normally have sinus arrhythmia, in which the heart rate increases with inspiration and decreases with expiration. If your patient can cooperate, ask him to hold his breath for a few seconds — his heart rate will become regular if he has sinus arrhythmia but will continue to be irregular if he has a true arrhythmia.

Tachycardia is a common response to such stressors as anxiety, fever, hypoxia, hypercapnia, and hypovolemia. In neonates, the response to hypoxemia is bradycardia; in older children, you'll note tachycardia. When the tachycardia can't fully compensate for the hypoxemia, tissue hypoxia and hypercapnia will develop with ensuing acidosis and bradycardia. A child in distress with bradycardia is displaying an ominous sign of impending cardiac arrest.

Normal pediatric vital signs

In children, normal pulse rate, respiratory rate, and blood pressure vary with age, as shown in the chart below.

AGE	PULSE RATE (beats/minute)	RESPIRATORY RATE (breaths/minute)	BLOOD PRESSURE	
			AVERAGE SYSTOLIC (mm Hg)	AVERAGE DIASTOLIC (mm Hg)
Neonate (1 to 28 days)	110 to 150	60	80	46
3 months	110 to 140	40	89	60
6 months	100 to 140	30	89	60
1 year	100 to 140	25	98	64
2 years	90 to 100	20	94	62
3 years	80 to 120	20	100	64
4 years	80 to 100	20	100	66
5 years	80 to 100	20	94	56
6 years	80 to 100	20	100	58
10 years	70 to 110	20	110	60

Respirations. In infants and young children, breathing is primarily diaphragmatic and thoracic excursion is minimal. As a result, you may find it easier to obtain the respiratory rate by observing abdominal rather than thoracic excursion. Also, infants' respiratory rates may vary periodically, changing every 15 to 30 seconds. To obtain an accurate count, try to assess an infant's respiratory rate for more than the usual 15 seconds. If possible, assess respirations for a full 60 seconds. You also need to be aware that a child's respiratory rate is more responsive than an adult's to illness, emotion, and exercise. In fact, with stress, the rate can double.

A pediatric patient's respiratory rate can provide valuable clues to life-threatening conditions. Quiet tachypnea — rapid respirations without signs of respiratory distress — can alert you to such problems as metabolic acidosis, diabetic ketoacidosis, inborn errors of metabolism, salicylate overdose, and renal insufficiency. Quiet tachypnea results from the body's attempt to maintain normal pH by increasing minute ventilation; this causes a compensatory respiratory alkalosis.

Acutely ill infants and children with slow respiratory rates require careful assessment. A decreasing respiratory rate is an ominous trend in such conditions as hypothermia and central nervous system depression. However, such a decrease may just indicate fatigue—especially in a patient whose respiratory rate was previously elevated.

Blood pressure. First, try to auscultate the patient's blood pressure. This may be difficult if he's under age 1. If so, use an electronic stethoscope, which gives you a more accurate reading. If an electronic stethoscope isn't available, determine the systolic pressure by palpating the radial artery and recording the reading at which you first feel a pulse.

Because children have a proportionately smaller blood volume, even seemingly minor injuries can produce significant blood loss, possibly leading to shock. And because shock can develop insidiously, careful monitoring and frequent assessments are necessary.

Keep in mind that hypotension is a late and often sudden sign of shock. A fall of even 10 mm Hg in systolic blood pressure warrants close observation. A young child can actually lose up to 25% of his total blood volume before hypotension becomes apparent. So you must closely observe for other signs in a potentially hypovolemic child. The best indicators of impending shock in such children include tachycardia, cold extremities in a warm environment, increased diastolic blood pressure, and delayed capillary refill time. In infants, a decreased heart rate and a weak pulse may be the only indications of impending shock.

Health history. During the health history interview, direct as many questions as possible to the child. Of course, with a young child, you'll have to rely on the parents to provide most of the information. But even a young child can discuss his symptoms to some degree and confirm the information his parents are giving you.

After asking about the chief complaint, be sure to explore any pertinent medical history. Possible topics include prenatal history and birth complications, congenital abnormalities, neonatal complications, developmental history, nutritional status, childhood illnesses, and immunizations.

Assessing elderly patients

When assessing an elderly patient, you'll use the same techniques you would for any other adult. However, you'll need to take into account the physiologic and biological changes that are a normal part of aging. Impaired respiratory and cardiovascular functions may make your patient more susceptible to airway, breathing, and circulation difficulties. And decreased function in other body systems may exacerbate the patient's current condition. An elderly patient also may have one or more chronic diseases.

Even though you need to consider age-related changes when assessing an elderly patient, make sure you avoid stereotypical misconceptions that may interfere with an accurate assessment. For example, not all elderly patients are frail, slow-moving, and sensory-impaired.

During your assessment, follow these broad guidelines:
• Stand or sit where the patient can see you as you speak to him.
• Be aware of common age-related visual difficulties.
• Speak clearly, distinctly, and slowly, in a well-modulated voice. (If necessary, consider turning your stethoscope around, placing the earpieces in the patient's ears, and talking into the diaphragm.)

General observations. An elderly patient may have several chronic health problems that can complicate the disorder underlying his chief complaint. An elderly patient's symptoms may also be nonspecific. For example, a patient who has an acute systemic infection or a cerebrovascular accident may show only one symptom—confusion. Because the brain is the most vulnerable organ in elderly patients, any new illness or physical problem is likely to cause a change in mental status. These changes can include confusion, agitation, and perhaps delirium.

When you assess your patient, also remember that he may have decreased function in all his body systems. Expect him to have slowed intestinal motility, diminished renal function, decreased sensation and reflexes, reduced muscle mass, and weakened bones and joints. A hip or pelvic fracture, for instance, may result from just a small amount of force.

Vital signs. An elderly patient will probably have reduced cardiac output (by as much as 35% in many patients over age 70), decreased arterial wall elasticity, and arterial and venous insufficiency. Such factors make an elderly person more likely than a younger one to have chronic heart disease, hypertension, and atherosclerosis.

The patient's peripheral pulses may be decreased if he has chronic venous and arterial insufficiency. So weak or absent peripheral pulses don't necessarily indicate shock or circulatory impairment in such a patient.

When assessing the patient's respirations, expect chest expansion to be decreased because of muscle weakness, general physical disability, a sedentary life-style, and possibly calcifications of the rib articulations.

To ensure an accurate reading, measure blood pressure in both arms. Evaluate the patient's pulse and blood pressure against what's normal for him. Because of increased vagal tone, an elderly patient may have a slower heart rate, although in some cases the heart rate becomes more rapid with age. Ectopic beats, fairly common in elderly patients, may produce irregularities in heart rhythm. If your patient has a sclerosed aorta, you may note an elevated systolic blood pressure with a normal diastolic pressure.

Health history. Help the patient focus on the most important aspects of his history. He'll probably have an extensive medical history—and difficulty relating it chronologically. Help him by asking questions that keep him on track. For example, you might ask if he had a particular illness, injury, or operation before or after his last birthday. Remember to keep your language simple and direct.

Modify the health history interview for an elderly patient if his cognitive or sensory function is diminished. Otherwise, focus on the same areas you would for any adult—but place special emphasis on medication use.

If possible, obtain a detailed medication history—including over-the-counter drugs. Make sure you ask how and when he takes his medications. In many cases, an elderly patient's chief complaint may result from noncompliance with a prescribed medication regimen, a drug interaction, or an overdose of medication (such as digitalis or an antiarrhythmic agent).

When exploring the chief complaint, remember that the patient's pain tolerance may be increased or his pain sensations diminished from sensory loss. Make sure you don't underestimate the severity of his chief complaint just because he doesn't report severe pain.

Be aware that your patient may hesitate to report symptoms because he attributes them to "old age" and feels that nothing can be done to ease them. The patient also may have adjusted to gradual changes and thus simply may not have noticed his symptoms.

Suggested readings

Engel, J. *Pocket Nurse Guide to Pediatric Assessment*. St. Louis: C.V. Mosby Co., 1989.

Kitt, S., and Kaiser, J., eds. *Emergency Nursing: A Physiologic and Clinical Perspective*. Philadelphia: W.B. Saunders Co., 1989.

Matteson, M.A., and McConnell, E.S. *Gerontological Nursing: Concepts & Practice*. Philadelphia: W.B. Saunders Co., 1988.

Morton, P.G. *Health Assessment in Nursing*. Springhouse, Pa.: Springhouse Corp., 1989.

Potter, P.A. *Pocket Nurse Guide to Physical Assessment*, 2nd ed. St. Louis: C.V. Mosby Co., 1990.

Raish, P., and Klaus, B.J. *Every Nurse's Guide to Physical Assessment: A Primary Care Focus*. New York: John Wiley & Sons, 1987.

Rea, R., et al., eds. *Emergency Nursing Core Curriculum*, 3rd ed. Philadelphia: W.B. Saunders Co., 1987.

4

ASSESSMENT
OF THE
HEAD AND NECK

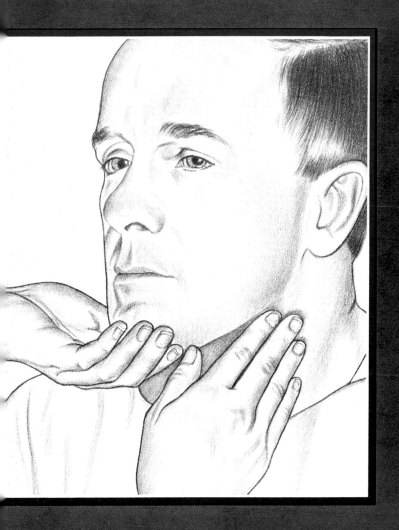

When a patient complains of head pain, he may have a simple tension headache. Or it may be a symptom of something more serious — a neurologic disorder, perhaps. To find out, explore his chief complaint by performing a systematic rapid assessment.

In this chapter, you'll review how to rapidly assess a headache and other common chief complaints of the head and neck. The chapter contains four sections — the first focuses on the head and neck as a whole, the other three focus on the nose and mouth, the eyes, and the ears, respectively. Each section begins with general observations you'll make and vital signs you'll check. Next comes the history questions you'll use to learn more about a particular chief complaint. Then you'll find an explanation of the physical assessment you'll perform, including inspection, palpation, and any further assessments you may need to make. Each section concludes with special considerations for assessing pediatric and elderly patients.

Three points to remember as you assess: First, when you're assessing one area of the body, be ready to move to another area if you need to gather additional information. For instance, you may need to move to the chest if your patient's complaint of dizziness leads you to suspect hypertension. Next, be prepared to interrupt your assessment and intervene if you detect anything that calls for immediate attention, such as severe bleeding. Finally, as you perform the physical assessment, focus on the areas most relevant to the chief complaint — inspecting the face for shape and symmetry takes on more importance when your patient complains of facial swelling, for example. But if possible, perform all the appropriate assessments to obtain a complete picture.

Head and neck

If your patient's chief complaint isn't specific to one area or structure of the head and neck — for instance, if he complains of a headache — your rapid assessment must focus on the entire head and neck. (See *Reviewing head and neck structures.*)

General observations
Begin your assessment by checking your patient's level of consciousness (LOC), overall appearance and body movements, facial expressions, and skin condition.

Level of consciousness. First, determine your patient's LOC, a key indicator of cerebral function. Often the first sign of a deteriorating neurologic condition, a decrease in LOC can alert you to a life-threatening problem. Be especially alert for a decreased LOC if your patient has a head injury or suffers from a condition that can alter blood flow and perfusion or increase intracranial pressure (ICP).

Overall appearance and body movements. Observe your patient's overall appearance. Note whether his head and neck are tilted, a possible sign of a neck muscle problem. Check too for signs of generalized head or neck trauma. If you see such signs, assume your patient has a cervical spine injury and immobilize the cervical spine immediately.

Facial expressions. Observe your patient's facial expression for clues

Reviewing head and neck structures

These two illustrations show the anatomic structures of the head and neck.

SKULL AND SURROUNDING STRUCTURES

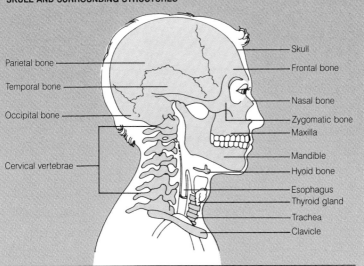

Parietal bone

Temporal bone

Occipital bone

Cervical vertebrae

Skull

Frontal bone

Nasal bone

Zygomatic bone

Maxilla

Mandible

Hyoid bone

Esophagus

Thyroid gland

Trachea

Clavicle

NECK MUSCLES AND LANDMARKS

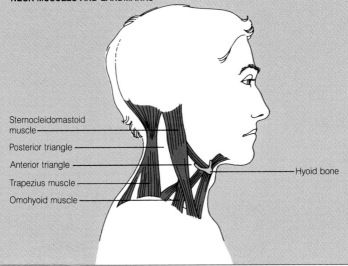

Sternocleidomastoid muscle

Posterior triangle

Anterior triangle

Trapezius muscle

Omohyoid muscle

Hyoid bone

to his mental and emotional status. Note any grimacing or other signs of discomfort. Watch carefully to see if he holds or rubs any part of his head, face, or neck.

Skin condition. Look for changes in skin color — pallor, jaundice, cyanosis — and note areas of obvious discoloration, such as bruises. Check for breaks in skin integrity, lesions, visible masses, swelling, and bleeding.

Vital signs
Measure your patient's pulse, respiratory rate, and blood pressure — important, although late, indicators of changing ICP and blood flow. Also check his temperature. In a patient with a severe head injury, you'll initially see a widening pulse pressure as ICP rises.

Suspect hypovolemic shock, which can alter cerebral blood flow and perfusion, if your patient's blood pressure falls below 80 mm Hg (or 30 mm Hg below his baseline) and he has a narrowed pulse pressure and a rapid, weak, or irregular pulse.

History
After completing your general observations, obtain a quick history of the patient's chief complaint. For the head and neck, such complaints include head injury, headache, dizziness, neck pain or stiffness, facial edema, and facial pain. Use critical questions to quickly gather the essential information.

Head injury. If your patient complains of a head injury, explore his problem by asking appropriate questions from this list.
• How did he hurt his head? Was he dizzy or did he have blurred vision beforehand? Determine whether he

was in a potentially hazardous situation, such as walking on a wet floor when he hurt himself.
• Did he lose consciousness when he hurt his head? If so, for how long?
• Has he gotten better or worse since he hurt his head?
• Find out if the patient is or was experiencing any other problems, such as neck pain, headache, vision problems, vomiting, loss of bowel or bladder control, or memory loss.
• Does he have a history of seizures or blackouts? If so, does he or did he take any medication for the problem?

Analyzing the chief complaint. Head injuries usually result from a fall or a blow to the head and can range from a minor concussion to a skull fracture or hematoma. Secondary responses — increased ICP, for instance — result as the body responds to the injury. A head injury may also change the shape of the skull, causing other abnormalities.

If a patient has had a previous head injury, he may initially complain of blurred vision or frequent headaches, not the injury itself. So when you hear these complaints, suspect such an injury.

Always treat a head injury patient as if he has a spinal cord injury until the possibility has been ruled out. Even if he claims his head injury is only minor, he may have contusions, a hematoma, or a skull fracture.

Headache. If your patient complains of a headache, explore his problem by asking appropriate questions from the list below. As you question the patient, observe him carefully, noting any discrepancies between his behavior and his description of the headache.
• When did he first notice the head-

ache? How often does it occur? Does he notice it at any particular time of day? Does it start slowly over a few hours or days or abruptly over a few minutes? How long does it last?
• Find out exactly where he feels the pain. On one or both sides, or all over his head?
• Have him describe the pain. Is it throbbing or shooting? Like a band of pressure? Sharp or dull?
• What relieves the headache? What makes it worse?
• Does he also have neck pain or stiffness? Do his arms, legs, hands, or feet feel numb or tingly?
• Ask if other symptoms, such as nausea or dizziness, precede the headache.

Analyzing the chief complaint.
Headaches rank as the most common neurologic symptom. About 90% of them are benign and result from vascular or muscle contractions or both (see *Comparing benign headaches,* page 52). Other causes include ocular and sinus disorders and the effects of drugs, treatments, and tests. But some pathologic headaches signal a severe neurologic disorder, such as increased ICP or meningeal irritation.

If your patient describes his headache as feeling like a band of pressure at the back of his head and says aspirin relieves the pain, the cause is probably a muscle contraction or tension. Vascular headaches — migraine or cluster headaches — produce throbbing, unilateral pain that analgesics don't relieve. Brain tumors cause intermittent, deep-seated, dull pain at the tumor site that the patient will feel most intensely in the mornings. And hypertension can cause a slightly throbbing occipital headache that the patient notices most when he wakes up.

Dizziness. If your patient complains of dizziness, explore his problem by asking appropriate questions from this list.
• What exactly does the patient mean by dizzy?
• When did the dizziness start? Has he had this dizziness before? How often and when? How long does it last? Find out what relieves the dizziness and what makes it worse.
• When the patient feels dizzy, does he also feel as if he's going to faint? Does he break into a heavy sweat or notice blurred or double vision, a headache, giddiness, or weakness?
• Ask if he has trouble sleeping or concentrating. Is he upset about anything?
• Does he have a history of hypertension or diabetes? Is he taking any medications? If so, what are they and how often does he take them?

Analyzing the chief complaint. Dizziness, a feeling of imbalance or faintness, can result from an inadequate blood flow and oxygen supply to the cerebrum. Your patient may also complain of giddiness, weakness, confusion, and blurred or double vision, but he shouldn't complain of a whirling sensation. If he does, he has vertigo, not dizziness. Episodes of dizziness usually pass quickly and range in severity from mild to moderate, with an abrupt or gradual onset. Standing up quickly can aggravate dizziness; lying down and resting may relieve the problem.

Simple anxiety can cause dizziness. But dizziness can also signal a more serious disorder. Respiratory and cardiovascular disorders, postconcussion syndromes, hypertension, and vertebrobasilar artery insufficiency all cause dizziness.

If your patient reports dizziness

Comparing benign headaches

As the chart shows, the two major types of benign headaches—muscle-contraction and vascular headaches—are quite different. In a combined headache, features of both appear. Treatment of a combined headache requires analgesics and sedatives.

CHARACTERISTIC	MUSCLE-CONTRACTION HEADACHES	VASCULAR HEADACHES
Incidence	• Most common type, accounting for 80% of all headaches	• More common in women and those with a family history of migraines • Onset after puberty
Precipitating factors	• Stress, anxiety, or tension • Prolonged muscle contraction without structural damage • Eye, ear, and paranasal sinus disorders that produce reflex muscle contractions	• Hormone fluctuations • Alcohol • Emotional upset • Too little or too much sleep • Foods and seasonings, such as chocolate, cheese, cured meats, and monosodium glutamate • Weather changes, such as shifts in barometric pressure
Intensity and duration	• Produce an aching tightness or a band of pain around the head, especially in the neck, occipital, and temporal areas • Occur frequently and usually last for several hours	• May begin with an awareness of an impending migraine or a 5- to 15-minute prodrome of neurologic deficits such as visual disturbances; tingling of the face, lips, or hands; dizziness; or unsteady gait • Produce severe, constant, throbbing pain that's typically unilateral and may be incapacitating • Last for 4 to 6 hours
Associated signs and symptoms	• Tense neck and facial muscles	• Anorexia, nausea, and vomiting • Occasionally, photophobia, sensitivity to loud noises, weakness, and fatigue • Depending on the type (cluster headache or classic, common, or hemiplegic migraine), patient may experience chills, depression, eye pain, ptosis, tearing, rhinorrhea, diaphoresis, and facial flushing
Alleviating factors	• Mild analgesics, muscle relaxants, or other drugs during an attack • Measures to reduce stress, such as biofeedback, relaxation techniques and counseling, and posture correction to prevent attacks	• Methysergide and propranolol to prevent onset • Ergot drugs at the first sign of a migraine • Rest in a quiet, darkened room • Elimination of irritating foods from diet

of varying intensity that lasts for a few seconds to 24 hours, triggered by turning his head to the side and accompanied by double vision, suspect a transient ischemic attack — often a signal of impending stroke.

Neck pain or stiffness. If your patient complains of neck pain or stiffness, explore his problem by asking appropriate questions from this list.
• When did the neck pain or stiffness start? How long has the patient had it?
• Have him describe the pain. Is it throbbing, sharp, or shooting? Does it radiate to the arms, shoulders, or hands or down the back? Is it constant or intermittent?
• Does a particular activity cause the pain or stiffness? Does moving his neck aggravate it? What makes it better or worse?
• Has he recently injured his head, back, or neck?

Analyzing the chief complaint. Neck pain and stiffness may originate in any neck structure, ranging from the meninges and cervical vertebrae to the neck's blood vessels, muscles, and lymphatic tissue. Or the problem can be referred from other areas of the body.

Causes can be relatively minor. A simple sprain can result in pain and tenderness and restrict the neck's range of motion; improper alignment can make the neck feel stiff. The pain can also stem from something more serious, such as trauma or degenerative, congenital, inflammatory, metabolic, or neoplastic disorders.

If you suspect the pain or stiffness results from trauma, immobilize the cervical spine at once.

Facial edema. If your patient com-

plains of facial swelling, explore his problem by asking appropriate questions from this list.
• When did the patient first notice the swelling? Has it gotten better or worse?
• Does he have any associated pain? If so, tell him to point to the area on his face that hurts.
• Determine if he's had an infection recently. If so, where was it located? Did he take any medication for it? If so, did he take all the medication prescribed?
• Ask if he's taking any other medications, such as steroids. How long has he been taking them?

Analyzing the chief complaint. Facial edema results from a disruption of the hydrostatic and osmotic pressures that govern fluid movement between the arteries, veins, and lymphatics. Edema may localize in one area — around the eyes, for instance — or it may cover a larger area, extending to the neck and upper arms. Occasionally painful, it may develop gradually or abruptly, and it sometimes precedes the onset of peripheral or generalized edema.

Facial swelling may be caused by a local problem, such as jaw swelling from an abscessed tooth or swelling from sinusitis or salivary gland cancer. Or the cause may be a systemic problem, such as nephrotic syndrome or prolonged use of steroids. Other systemic causes of facial edema include venous, inflammatory, and some systemic disorders; trauma; malnutrition; allergies; and the effects of drugs, tests, and treatments.

Watch swelling caused by burns or an allergic reaction closely; such swelling could cut off your patient's airway. Make sure you assess his respiratory status and maintain his airway and breathing.

Head and neck: Normal findings

Inspection
Normal findings include:
☐ a symmetrical, lesion-free skull
☐ symmetrical facial structures with no cyanosis or vascular lesions
☐ unrestricted range of motion in the neck
☐ an ability to shrug shoulders, a sign of adequately functioning cranial nerve XI (accessory nerve)
☐ no bulging of the thyroid
☐ symmetrical, unswollen lymph nodes.

Palpation
Normal findings include:
☐ no lumps or tenderness on the head
☐ symmetrical strength in the face muscles, a sign of adequately functioning cranial nerves V and VII (trigeminal and facial nerves)
☐ symmetrical sensation when you stroke a wisp of cotton on each cheek
☐ mobile, soft lymph nodes less than ½" (1 cm) in size with no tenderness
☐ symmetrical pulses in the carotid arteries
☐ a palpable, symmetrical, lesion-free thyroid and no thyroid tenderness
☐ the trachea at midline position and no tracheal tenderness
☐ no crepitus, tenderness, or lesions in the cervical spine
☐ symmetrical muscle strength in the neck.

Facial pain. If your patient complains of facial pain, explore his problem by asking appropriate questions from this list.
• When did the pain start? What was he doing when it began? Has he ever had the pain before? How long did it last?
• Have the patient point to where he feels the pain and describe it. Is it stabbing, throbbing, or dull?
• What relieves the pain? What makes it worse?
• Has he recently suffered a head injury or had an infection? What about recent dental work?

Analyzing the chief complaint. Typically paroxysmal and intense, facial pain most often occurs along the pathway of a specific nerve branch, usually cranial nerve V (the trigeminal nerve). Several neurologic, vascular, and infectious disorders lead to facial pain. It can also be referred from the ear, nose, sinuses, teeth, neck, or jaw. Most commonly, facial pain results from trigeminal neuralgia.

Question your patient carefully about the nature and location of his pain. He may have trouble differentiating facial pain from the more diffuse pain of headache.

Physical assessment
While performing your physical assessment, keep in mind the basic anatomy of the head and neck and the normal assessment findings. (See *Head and neck: Normal findings*.) To rapidly assess the head and neck, you'll mainly use inspection and palpation, although you also need to auscultate the neck to assess blood flow and tracheal breath sounds. Before you begin, have your patient sit up, if possible, so you can examine all sides of his head.

Inspection. Carefully inspect your patient's head and neck, making sure all structures are intact and have no visible deformities.

Head. Note your patient's expression. A distorted expression may result from facial swelling, injury, or pain. Some expressions may even point to specific disorders. A patient with Parkinson's disease, for instance, may stare blankly. And a startled gaze can be normal, but it can also result from hyperthyroidism.

Next, inspect the size, shape, and contour of your patient's head. Note any asymmetry or deformity, possibly the result of trauma (although surgical removal of part of the skull can also cause deformity). Look for indentations in the skull, a possible sign of a depressed fracture. A swollen, ecchymotic area may be the only sign of a linear fracture. Check the scalp and hair, looking for any lesions, abrasions, lacerations, swelling, or bleeding.

Move on to the face, noting color, shape, and symmetry. Asymmetry and distortion can result from facial edema or a cranial nerve problem. But if you see periorbital and facial edema accompanied by cyanosis of the lips, suspect congestive heart failure (CHF). Periorbital edema can also point to renal failure. Check whether the eyes are equidistant and if they align horizontally with the outer rim of the ears. Look for facial lesions, rashes, swelling, and redness. Note any tics, twitching, or other abnormal movement that may signal a nerve problem.

Neck. After you've looked at the patient's head, inspect his neck for edema, masses, or scars. Note any asymmetry. Look for pulsations in the jugular veins, which can signal such disorders as CHF, cardiac tamponade, and hypervolemia. Check for jugular vein distention by noting the height of the jugular vein's pulsations above the angle of Louis

(you'll need to place your patient in the semi-Fowler's position to do this).

If the patient's condition permits, ask him to move his head and neck through the entire range of motion and shrug his shoulders. Look for signs of pain and stiffness, which may stem from several disorders, including trauma, cervical arthritis, and osteoporosis. You may also note muscle spasm and tenderness — the results of simple tension or a neck injury that doesn't involve the vertebrae.

Inspect the lymph nodes, noting size and symmetry. Enlarged lymph nodes may indicate a local or systemic infection, although a past infection, if serious enough, may have left them permanently enlarged. (See *Locating the lymph nodes,* page 56.)

Palpation. Now, palpate your patient's head and neck to gather further information. Use your fingertips to feel skin textures and the pads of your fingers to assess the configuration of bony structures and skin lesions.

Head. First, palpate the contour and symmetry of the head and scalp, using a gentle rotary motion. If you feel any lacerations that you missed during inspection, apply a dressing to control bleeding, if necessary.

With both hands, palpate your patient's face bilaterally to assess skin tone and facial contour. To check facial muscle tone, assess the cheeks for recoil. Test the function of cranial nerve VII (the facial nerve) by simultaneously palpating the muscles on both sides of your patient's face as the patient smiles, frowns, grits his teeth, and puffs out his cheeks.

Next, palpate the temporal pulses

Locating the lymph nodes

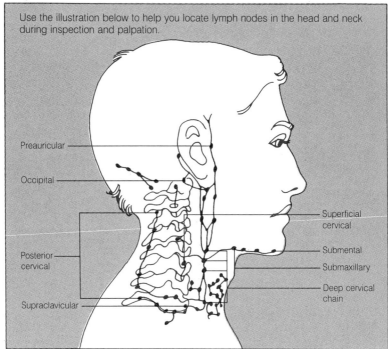

Use the illustration below to help you locate lymph nodes in the head and neck during inspection and palpation.

Preauricular

Occipital

Superficial cervical

Submental

Posterior cervical

Submaxillary

Deep cervical chain

Supraclavicular

for strength and rhythm. Then check the temporomandibular joints for movement and alignment. Note any signs of discomfort. (See *Palpating the temporomandibular joints*.)

Neck. As you move down to the neck, palpate the chain of lymph nodes, assessing size, shape, mobility, consistency, and tenderness. Compare one side with the other. You'll often find enlarged lymph nodes in a patient who complains of facial pain or swelling or neck pain and stiffness.

Next, palpate the carotid arteries to assess the character of the pulse. Abnormalities in rate or rhythm

point to a diminished cerebral blood flow. If you note thrills, a sign of turbulent blood flow, suspect atherosclerosis of the carotid artery or aortic valve disease. Remember, check the arteries one at a time; if you palpate both at the same time, you could trigger severe bradycardia. And don't massage the carotid sinus—located at the bifurcation of the carotid arteries; the resulting bradycardia could lead to cardiac arrest.

If you suspect a thyroid problem, palpate the thyroid by standing behind your patient and placing your hands around his neck, with the fingertips of both hands over the lower trachea. Ask the patient to swallow as you feel for the thyroid isthmus. Lying across the trachea just below the cricoid cartilage, the thyroid isthmus rises with swallowing. Then feel for enlargement or nodules on the butterfly lobes, attached to either side of the isthmus.

Check the position of the trachea by palpating the space between it and the sternocleidomastoid muscle. A narrowing on either side means the trachea has deviated to that side, probably from a mass in the neck or mediastinum or a pulmonary problem. (See *Palpating the trachea,* page 58.)

Finally, palpate down the back of the neck over the bony prominences of the cervical vertebrae, checking for signs of swelling, pain, and tenderness. Then feel either side of the prominences to check alignment.

Auscultation. With the bell of the stethoscope, listen over the major blood vessels in the patient's neck, particularly the carotid artery. Be sure to place only light pressure on the bell. Start at the base of the neck and move up toward the jaw. Ask your patient to hold his breath while you listen so his breath sounds don't interfere with the sounds of circulation. Listen for bruits — evidence of turbulent blood flow. If you hear them toward the base of the neck, suspect cardiac vessel disease; those heard near the jaw usually result from a disorder of cranial circulation.

Further assessment. Signs and symptoms affecting the head and neck often result from a disorder in another part of the body — sometimes a life-threatening disorder. So be ready to expand your physical assessment. If your patient has a head or neck injury or complains of

Palpating the temporomandibular joints

To palpate the temporomandibular joints — located just in front of and slightly below the auricles — place your hands on either side of the patient's face. Cover the temporomandibular joints with your middle three fingers. Then press gently as the patient opens and closes her mouth, assessing for mobility, discomfort, and crepitus.

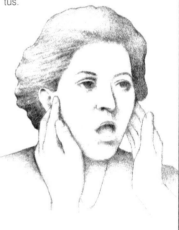

neck pain and stiffness, for instance, you'll need to assess the extremities for paresthesia, paralysis, and muscle function. Or if you note jugular vein pulsations or an abnormal cardiac pulse, you'll need to immediately proceed with a cardiac assessment.

Because the head and neck house the respiratory center, you may need to move to the lungs and respiratory structures if you suspect a respiratory problem. You also may need to assess the lungs for a tension pneumothorax if you note tracheal deviation.

After obtaining a history and performing the physical assessment,

Palpating the trachea

Face the patient and place your thumbs on either side of his trachea above the suprasternal notch. Then gently slide both thumbs at the same speed out along the upper edge of the clavicle until you reach the sterno-cleidomastoid muscle. Your thumbs should travel an equal distance; if they don't, the trachea has deviated from the midline.

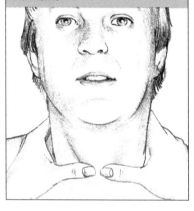

you'll begin to form a diagnostic impression. (See *Head and neck: Interpreting your findings.*)

Pediatric considerations

When you assess a child's head and neck, certain assessment techniques and findings will vary, depending on his developmental stage.

Head. When assessing a neonate, keep in mind that premature closing of the sutures or molding during vaginal delivery may have altered the shape of his head and face. You may also notice slight asymmetry in an infant's head caused by his always sleeping in the same position. And remember to palpate a child's parotid gland to check for the enlargement associated with mumps.

Head circumference. For a child under age 2, measure the circumference of his head. Record your measurement in centimeters and compare it with the normal range for a child of his age. Report an abnormal finding.

Fontanels. For a child under age 2, you'll assess the fontanels. Before doing so, sit him upright and try to keep him calm and quiet. Then inspect the area, particularly the large anterior fontanel. The fontanels should look almost flush with the scalp surface, and you should see slight pulsations.

Next, gently palpate the fontanels, using the pads of your index and middle fingers. The fontanels should feel soft and either flat or slightly indented. Palpate the sutures, too, which should feel smooth. They shouldn't feel as if they're separated or overriding each other.

Neck. You'll have to perform passive range-of-motion exercises to assess a young child's neck muscles. Insufficiently developed neck muscles keep a child under 2 weeks from turning his head; a child under 2 months from lifting his head more than 90 degrees when prone; and a child less than about 3 months from holding his head upright while seated. Keep in mind, too, that a child may normally have a number of small, firm, palpable lymph nodes in his neck.

Geriatric considerations

An elderly patient typically has wrinkled skin on his face because of an overall reduction in subcutaneous fat. In a thin patient, you may be able to see the temporal artery under the forehead skin.

Tell an elderly patient to move his

Head and neck: Interpreting your findings

After you assess the patient, a group of findings may lead you to suspect a particular disorder. The chart below shows you some common groups of findings for the chief complaints of the head and neck, along with the appropriate nursing diagnostic categories and probable causes.

CHIEF COMPLAINT AND FINDINGS	NURSING DIAGNOSTIC CATEGORIES	PROBABLE CAUSE
Head injury		
• Agitation • Confusion • Decreased level of consciousness (LOC) progressing from drowsiness to coma • Focal neurologic deficits such as hemiparesis • Headache	• Altered cerebral tissue perfusion • Fear • Potential for further injury	Subdural hematoma
• Recent history of hitting head during a fall • Decreased LOC • Dizziness • Projectile vomiting • Pulse and respirations decreased from baseline	• Altered cerebral tissue perfusion • Fear • Pain • Potential for further injury • Potential for impaired gas exchange	Skull fracture
Headache		
• Pain localized to occipital region • Worsening of pain on awakening and lessening of pain as day goes on • Altered LOC • Blurred vision • Confusion • Diastolic blood pressure greater than 120 mm Hg • Nausea and vomiting • S_4 heart sound • Restlessness • Seizures	• Knowledge deficit • Pain • Potential for injury	Hypertension
• Anxiety • No history of recent head trauma • Tense face and neck muscles	• Altered role performance • Anxiety • Pain	Benign muscle-contraction headache

(continued)

DIAGNOSTIC IMPRESSION

Head and neck: Interpreting your findings (continued)

CHIEF COMPLAINT AND FINDINGS	NURSING DIAGNOSTIC CATEGORIES	PROBABLE CAUSE
Dizziness		
• Dizziness triggered by turning head • Confusion • Decreased LOC • Dysarthria • Dysphagia • Pallor • Paresis and numbness • Ptosis • Unilateral or bilateral diplopia, blindness, or visual field deficits • Vomiting and hiccups	• Altered cerebral tissue perfusion • Potential for injury • Potential for trauma • Visual and auditory sensory-perceptual alterations	Cerebrovascular accident
• Apprehension • Diaphoresis • Pallor • Respiratory rate of 30 breaths/minute • Shortness of breath	• Altered cardiopulmonary tissue perfusion • Altered cerebral tissue perfusion • Anxiety • Impaired gas exchange • Ineffective breathing pattern	Hyperventilation syndrome
Neck pain or stiffness		
• Sudden, severe onset of pain • Nuchal rigidity • Fever • Nausea and vomiting • Positive Brudzinski's sign • Positive Kernig's sign	• Altered cerebral tissue perfusion • Hyperthermia • Knowledge deficit	Bacterial meningitis
Facial edema		
• Periorbital edema • Peripheral dependent edema • Lethargy • Nausea • Pallor • Weight gain	• Altered renal tissue perfusion • Fatigue • Fluid volume excess	Nephrotic syndrome
• Edema most severe around eyes • Facial erythema • Facial urticaria • Patient taking ampicillin	• Anxiety • Body image disturbance • Knowledge deficit • Potential for fluid volume deficit	Allergic reaction
Facial pain		
• Pain triggered by temperature extremes, facial movement, or touching nose, mouth, or cheek • Paroxysmal, intense pain	• Altered nutrition: Less than body requirements • Pain	Trigeminal neuralgia

head slowly and carefully to avoid pain when you assess range of motion. Many elderly patients have a decreased range of motion and neck pain from osteoporosis or arthritis.

Nose and mouth

When a patient has a complaint related to the nose or mouth — such as a nosebleed or a sore throat — you'll need to focus your rapid assessment on these structures. (See *Reviewing nose and mouth structures,* pages 62 and 63.)

General observations
Begin by looking at the overall appearance of the nose and mouth, particularly the nostrils and lips. If you notice nasal flaring, your patient could have a respiratory problem; a drooping mouth could point to a neurologic impairment.

Then look at the skin surrounding his nose and mouth, noting the color of his lips and the area immediately surrounding his mouth. Any discoloration or break in skin integrity could signal a problem. Note any swelling, bleeding, or drainage.

Next, listen to your patient's voice, noting the tone and listening for hoarseness or a nasal quality. Observe for dentures or any missing teeth. Smell his breath to detect any unusual odors.

Vital signs
Check the patient's vital signs, especially his temperature. A fever indicates infection, a common problem with complaints of the nose and mouth. If you notice any sign of injury or if your patient has a nosebleed, pay close attention to his pulse rate and blood pressure.

History
After completing your general observations and vital signs check, obtain a quick history of the patient's chief complaint. For the nose and mouth, such complaints include nasal stuffiness and discharge, throat pain, epistaxis, and dysphagia. Use critical questions to quickly gather the essential information.

Nasal stuffiness and discharge. If your patient complains of nasal stuffiness or discharge or both, explore his problem by asking appropriate questions from this list.
● When did he first notice the problem? When does the stuffiness and discharge occur? Is it intermittent or continuous?
● Is one side worse than the other? Does he find himself breathing through his mouth? What relieves the problem? What makes it worse?
● Determine the color and amount of the discharge.
● Does he have pain along with the stuffiness or discharge?
● Has he had any nasal surgery or an injury to his nose? When?
● Does he take any medications? If so, what kind and how often?

Analyzing the chief complaint. Rarely serious problems, nasal stuffiness and discharge involve an obstruction of the nasal mucous membranes and a discharge of thin nasal mucus. Either self-limiting or chronic, these signs can result from systemic disorders; nasal or sinus disorders, such as a deviated septum; trauma, such as a basilar skull or nasal fracture; sinus or cranial surgery; excessive use of vasoconstricting nose drops or sprays; allergies; or an irritant such as tobacco smoke, dust, or fumes.

The nature of the disorder deter-

(Text continues on page 64.)

ANATOMY

Reviewing nose and mouth structures

These illustrations show the anatomic structures of the nose and mouth.

NOSE AND MOUTH

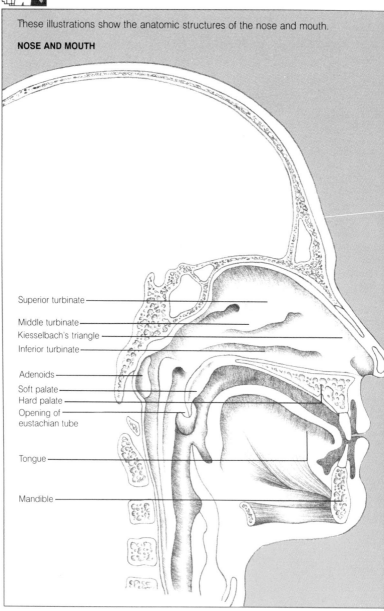

Superior turbinate

Middle turbinate

Kiesselbach's triangle

Inferior turbinate

Adenoids

Soft palate

Hard palate

Opening of eustachian tube

Tongue

Mandible

SINUSES

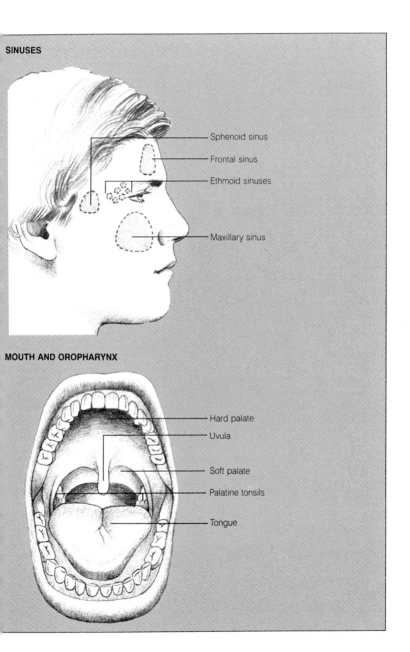

Sphenoid sinus
Frontal sinus
Ethmoid sinuses

Maxillary sinus

MOUTH AND OROPHARYNX

Hard palate
Uvula

Soft palate

Palatine tonsils

Tongue

mines what the nasal discharge looks like: bloody, clear, purulent, or serosanguineous. Bloody discharge usually results from something as simple as the patient blowing his nose too often, but spontaneous or traumatic epistaxis can cause such a discharge, too. Clear, thin drainage may simply point to rhinitis, or it may be cerebrospinal fluid (CSF) leaking from a basilar skull fracture. Thick white, yellow, or greenish drainage suggests an infection.

Throat pain. If your patient complains of throat pain, explore his problem by asking appropriate questions from this list.
• When did the throat pain start? Find out if he's had this kind of pain before.
• Is the pain constant or intermittent? On one or both sides? What relieves the pain or makes it worse?
• Does he have any associated problems — fever, ear pain, difficulty swallowing?
• Determine whether he's been near anyone else who had a cold or sore throat.

Analyzing the chief complaint. Throat pain — discomfort in any part of the pharynx — can range from a sensation of scratchiness to severe pain. It's often accompanied by ear pain because cranial nerves IX and X (the glossopharyngeal and vagus nerves) innervate the pharynx as well as the external ear.

Throat pain may result from infection, trauma, allergy, neoplasms, and certain systemic disorders. Such pain may also follow surgery and endotracheal intubation. Nonpathologic causes include dry mucous membranes associated with mouth breathing and laryngeal irritation resulting from vocal strain, alcohol consumption, and inhaling smoke or

chemicals like ammonia.

Epistaxis. If your patient has a nosebleed, explore his problem by asking appropriate questions from this list.
• When did the bleeding start? What was he doing when it started? Does anything relieve the nosebleed or make it worse?
• Ask if the patient has had nosebleeds before. If so, how often and when? Was the bleeding from one nostril or both? Was the bleeding heavy? Did it go on for a long time?
• Was the nose recently injured? Does he have a history of hypertension, bleeding disorder, or liver disease?
• Does he take any medications — particularly aspirin or anticoagulant drugs like warfarin? How much and how often?

Analyzing the chief complaint. Most nosebleeds occur in the anterior-inferior nasal septum, but they can also occur at the point where the inferior turbinates meet the nasopharynx. Usually unilateral, nosebleeds may seem bilateral when blood from the bleeding side runs behind the nasal septum and out the opposite side. Epistaxis ranges from mild oozing to severe, possibly life-threatening, blood loss.

Because the nose contains a rich supply of fragile blood vessels, anything from a simple infection to nasal trauma can cause bleeding. Other causes include hypertension (which can produce extreme epistaxis); air moving through and drying out the mucous membranes; certain drugs and treatments; and hematologic, coagulation, renal, and GI disorders.

Keep in mind that epistaxis can be life-threatening; you may need to interrupt your assessment and intervene to control the bleeding.

Dysphagia. If your patient has trouble swallowing, explore his problem by asking appropriate questions from this list.
• When did he first have trouble swallowing? How long has he had the problem? What was he doing when it started?
• Does it hurt to swallow? If so, is the pain constant or intermittent? Find out which phase of swallowing causes the most trouble. Does he, for instance, have the most trouble when he first tries to swallow?
• Does eating make the problem better or worse? Does he have more trouble swallowing solids or liquids? If liquids are the problem, does the temperature of the liquid have any effect?
• Does he have any other symptoms, such as vomiting, weight loss, hoarseness, shortness of breath, or a cough?

Analyzing the chief complaint. Classified by the phase of swallowing that's affected, dysphagia can be constant or intermittent. (See *Classifying dysphagia,* page 66.) Factors that can interfere with swallowing include severe pain, obstruction, abnormal peristalsis, an impaired gag reflex, and excessive, scanty, or thick oral secretions. The most common — sometimes the only — symptom of an esophageal disorder, dysphagia can also result from oropharyngeal, respiratory, neurologic, or collagen disorders and from certain toxins and treatments. Dysphagia can lead to malnutrition and dehydration and increases the risk of choking and aspiration.

Remember, dysphagia can be life-threatening. If your patient has a dysphagic attack and shows signs of respiratory distress, suspect an airway obstruction and prepare to deliver abdominal thrusts.

Physical assessment
As you perform your physical assessment, keep in mind the basic anatomy of the nose and mouth, along with the normal assessment findings. (See *Nose and mouth: Normal findings,* page 67.)

To rapidly assess the nose and mouth, you'll mainly use inspection and palpation, although you may need to use percussion to gather additional information. Before you begin, ask your patient to sit upright. Work in a well-lighted area and try to stand directly in front of him while you perform the assessment.

Inspection. Begin your physical assessment by carefully inspecting your patient's nose and mouth.

Nose. Inspect your patient's nose for symmetry, noting any deformity, swelling, or discoloration. Have him tilt his head back so you can check for septal deviation. Look for marked nasal flaring, a sign of respiratory distress. (Slight nasal flaring is normal.)

Next, look for drainage from the nostrils, observing its character for clues to its cause. Then assess the frontal and maxillary sinuses by inspecting the skin above and on either side of the nose for inflammation and edema. Swelling over the sinuses points to congestion and possible infection. Using a penlight, inspect the nostrils. Note any swelling, drainage, abnormal color, or signs of recent bleeding.

Mouth. After inspecting the nose, check the symmetry, texture, contour, and color of your patient's lips. If they look blue, suspect hypoxia; the patient will probably need oxy-

Classifying dysphagia

Swallowing occurs in three distinct phases, and dysphagia can be classified by the phase that it affects. Each phase suggests a specific pathology for dysphagia.

Phase 1
Swallowing begins in the *transfer phase* (shown in gray) with chewing and moistening of food with saliva. The tongue presses against the hard palate to transfer the chewed food to the back of the throat; cranial nerve V (trigeminal nerve) then stimulates the swallowing reflex. Phase 1 dysphagia typically results from a neuromuscular disorder.

Phase 2
In the *transport phase* (shown in light brown), the soft palate closes against the pharyngeal wall to prevent nasal regurgitation. At the same time, the larynx rises and the vocal cords close to keep food out of the lungs; breathing stops momentarily as the throat muscles constrict to move food into the esophagus. Phase 2 dysphagia usually indicates spasm or carcinoma.

Phase 3
Peristalsis and gravity work together in the *entrance phase* (shown in orange) to move food through the esophageal sphincter and into the stomach. Phase 3 dysphagia results from lower esophageal narrowing by diverticula, esophagitis, and other disorders.

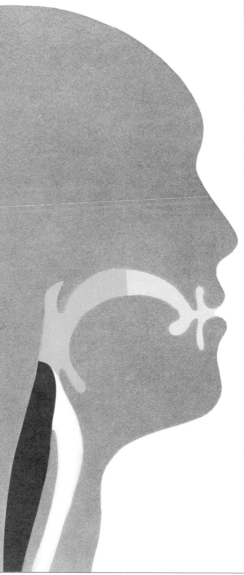

Nose and mouth: Normal findings

Inspection
Normal findings include:
☐ a symmetrical, lesion-free nose with no deviation of the septum or discharge
☐ little or no nasal flaring
☐ nonedematous frontal and maxillary sinuses
☐ an ability to identify familiar odors
☐ pinkish red nasal mucosa with no visible lesions and no purulent drainage
☐ no evidence of foreign bodies or dried blood in the nose
☐ pink lips with no dryness, cracking, lesions, or cyanosis
☐ symmetrical facial structures
☐ an ability to purse the lips and puff out the cheeks, a sign of an adequately functioning cranial nerve VII (facial nerve)
☐ an ability to easily open and close the mouth
☐ light pink, moist oral mucosa with no ulcers or lesions
☐ visible salivary ducts with no inflammation
☐ a white hard palate
☐ a pink soft palate
☐ pink gums with no tartar, inflammation, or hemorrhage
☐ all teeth intact with no signs of occlusion, caries, or breakage
☐ a pink tongue with no swelling, coating, ulcers, or lesions
☐ a tongue that moves easily and without tremor, a sign of a properly functioning cranial nerve XII (hypoglossal nerve)
☐ no swelling or inflammation on anterior and posterior arches
☐ no lesions or inflammation on posterior pharynx
☐ lesion-free tonsils that are the right size for the patient's age
☐ a uvula that moves when the patient says "ah" and a gag reflex when you touch a tongue blade to the posterior pharynx, signs of properly functioning cranial nerves IX and X.

Palpation
Normal findings include:
☐ no structural deviation, tenderness, or swelling in the external nose
☐ no tenderness or edema on the frontal and maxillary sinuses
☐ lips free from pain and induration
☐ no lesions, unusual color, tenderness, or swelling on the posterior and lateral surfaces of the tongue
☐ no tenderness, nodules, or swelling on the floor of the mouth.

gen. Note any lesions, fissures, or edema. Dry, cracked lips may signal a febrile illness, although cracking, especially at the corners of the mouth, can also result from vitamin B_6 deficiency, poor hygiene, or breathing dry air.

Using a gloved finger or tongue blade, pull back your patient's lips and check the color, texture, and hydration of his mucosa. (You may want to use a penlight to help you see.) Note any lesions. Then pull back his cheek and examine his buccal mucosa. Ask him to tilt his head back, so you can inspect the hard and soft palates. If the mucosa look red, suspect infection; if they look blue, suspect hypoxia. Ulcerations on the mucosa point to infection or poor nutrition, and thickened white patches—leukoplakia—may be precancerous.

Next, look closely at the gingivae, noting any marginal redness, edema, retraction, or bleed-

Eliciting a gag reflex

Before you check your patient's gag reflex, be sure to depress his tongue with a tongue blade. That way, you'll be able to see his pharynx clearly. Once you have his tongue depressed, touch a cotton-tipped applicator to each side of the posterior pharynx.

ing — signs of gingivitis. Note the number and appearance of the teeth.

Ask your patient to relax and stick out his tongue. Inspect its color, size, and position, noting any lesions or coating. Don't forget to check the underside. Then have him move his tongue up and down and sideways so you can evaluate the function of cranial nerve XII (the hypoglossal nerve). Note any deviation of the tongue to one side or the other.

While depressing the patient's tongue with a tongue blade, ask him to tilt his head back, open his mouth, and say "ah." Using a penlight, inspect the pharynx, noting any abnormal color, inflammation, edema, or exudate. Then examine the tonsils, uvula, soft palate, and posterior pharynx. If you notice the uvula deviating to one side when the patient says "ah," suspect a problem with the innervation of cranial nerve IX or X.

Next, evaluate your patient's gag reflex (see *Eliciting a gag reflex*). Like a deviated uvula, an absent gag reflex points to a problem with cranial nerve IX or X. An absent gag reflex also increases your patient's risk of aspiration.

Palpation. After inspection, palpate your patient's nose and mouth to gather further information.

Nose. Palpate the nose, checking for any painful or tender areas, swelling, displacement, or deformities you may not have noted on inspection. Tenderness with edema may indicate a fracture. Check the patency of each nostril by gently occluding one nostril and asking the patient to breathe out of the other. Then palpate the frontal and maxillary sinuses for inflammation and edema.

Mouth. To evaluate the muscle tone and surface structures of the mouth, gently pull the upper lip down, release it, and watch how it snaps back; then pull the lower lip up, and repeat the procedure. Assess the patient's tongue by grasping it with a gauze pad and moving it from side to side.

After obtaining a history and performing the physical assessment, you'll begin to form a diagnostic impression. (See *Nose and mouth: Interpreting your findings.*)

Pediatric considerations
When examining a child's nose and mouth, you need to be aware of certain variations in the normal findings.

Nose. When you assess an infant, remember his nose has a slightly flattened bridge. Keep in mind, too, that most infants younger than 6 months don't yet breathe through their mouths.

You won't palpate the frontal and maxillary sinuses of a child under age 8 because they haven't developed. If you notice nasal discharge on only one side or detect a strange odor, the child may have a foreign object stuck in his nose.

DIAGNOSTIC IMPRESSION

Nose and mouth: Interpreting your findings

After you assess the patient, a group of findings may lead you to suspect a particular disorder. The chart below shows you some common groups of findings for the chief complaints of the nose and mouth, along with the appropriate nursing diagnostic categories and probable causes.

CHIEF COMPLAINT AND FINDINGS	NURSING DIAGNOSTIC CATEGORIES	PROBABLE CAUSE
Nasal stuffiness and discharge		
• Purulent rhinorrhea • Cough • Fever • Headache • Malaise • Red swollen nasal mucosa • Sinus pain • Sore throat • Tenderness and swelling beneath eyebrows or on cheeks	• Hyperthermia • Olfactory sensory-perceptual alterations • Potential for infection	Sinusitis
• Blocked feeling in ears • Fatigue • Fever • Malaise • Myalgia • Normal breath sounds • Pulse regular but slightly elevated over baseline • Sneezing	• Ineffective airway clearance • Ineffective breathing patterns • Sensory-perceptual alterations • Sleep pattern disturbance	Common cold
Throat pain		
• Unilateral throat pain • Arthralgia • Dysphagia and odynophagia • Exudate • Fever • Headache • Malaise • Myalgia • Redness of one or both tonsillar pillars • Redness of oropharynx • Tender cervical lymph nodes on palpation	• Altered nutrition: Less than body requirements • Hyperthermia • Impaired swallowing • Pain	Bacterial tonsillitis
• Cough • Fever and chills • Headache • Malaise • Muscle aches • Weakness	• Altered nutrition: Less than body requirements • Hyperthermia • Impaired swallowing • Pain • Potential for infection	Influenza

(continued)

DIAGNOSTIC IMPRESSION

Nose and mouth: Interpreting your findings *(continued)*

CHIEF COMPLAINT AND FINDINGS	NURSING DIAGNOSTIC CATEGORIES	PROBABLE CAUSE
Epistaxis		
• Bilateral bleeding • Crepitation of nasal bones • Nasal deformity and displacement • Pain • Periorbital ecchymoses and edema	• Anxiety • Impaired tissue integrity (of the nasal mucosa) • Ineffective airway clearance • Olfactory sensory-perceptual alterations • Pain	Nasal fracture
• Unilateral bleeding • Long history of frequent mild nosebleeds • No bruising or accompanying bleeding apparent • Normal vital signs	• Anxiety • Impaired tissue integrity (of the nasal mucosa) • Knowledge deficit	Spontaneous epistaxis
Dysphagia		
• Dysarthria • Dyspnea • Emotional lability • Fasciculations • Muscle weakness and atrophy • Shallow respirations • Tachypnea	• Altered nutrition: Less than body requirements • Impaired swallowing • Potential for aspiration • Potential for injury • Self care deficit	Amyotrophic lateral sclerosis
• Worsening of dysphagia on lying down or stooping • Recent history of dysphagia associated with heartburn • Frequent belching • Frequent flatulence • Halitosis	• Altered nutrition: Less than body requirements • Impaired swallowing • Knowledge deficit	Hiatal hernia

Mouth. When you assess an infant's mouth, check for the sucking reflex by lightly touching his lips. As you look inside his mouth, you may notice raised white spots, called Epstein's pearls, along the gum line or on the hard palate. These usually disappear a few weeks after birth. You may also notice sucking lesions on the buccal membrane, another normal finding in infants. When examining any child's mouth, keep in mind that an abnormally large or small tongue may indicate a congenital abnormality.

You can assess an infant's oropharynx when he's crying, or use a tongue blade to open his mouth. Ask an older child to stick out his tongue as far as he can and pant so you can examine his posterior pharynx and tonsils. Remember, tonsils that look disproportionately small in an infant don't point to an abnormality. Tonsils are small in an infant. They increase in size until a child reaches adolescence and then shrink to normal adult size.

Geriatric considerations

In an elderly patient, you'll probably find some gingival recession and inflammation, along with missing or loose teeth. He may also have a dry mouth—the result of the decreased salivary production that occurs with aging—which can interfere with chewing and cause the mucosa to break down. You may also notice longitudinal or latitudinal fissures on his tongue, a normal occurrence with aging.

Eyes

When a patient has a complaint related to the eyes, such as eye pain or photophobia, perform your rapid assessment as described below. (See *Reviewing eye structures,* pages 72 and 73.)

General observations

Begin your assessment by looking at the overall appearance of the eyes, including the eyebrows, eyelids, eyelashes, and eyeballs. Note any asymmetry or gross abnormalities, such as ptosis. Look for redness, crusting, or excessive tearing. Observe whether the patient wears contact lenses or glasses. Then look at the skin color around his eyes and compare it with the rest of his facial skin, noting any signs of trauma.

Next, observe the patient's gaze, noting any distortions or deviations. Check his near vision by asking him

to read a sentence or two from a newspaper or identify an object in a picture. Check his distance vision by asking him to read the top lines of an eye chart or to read a newspaper headline on the other side of the room. You can also check distance vision by standing on the other side of the room and asking him to count the number of fingers you hold up. Assess his color perception by asking him to identify the color of a piece of clothing.

History

After completing your general observations, obtain a quick history of the patient's chief complaint. For the eyes, such complaints include eye pain, eye discharge, visual changes, diplopia, and photophobia. Use critical questions to gather the essential information.

Eye pain. If your patient complains of eye pain, explore his problem by asking appropriate questions from this list.
• When did the pain start? Did it come on suddenly or gradually? How long has the patient had the pain? Has he had it before?
• Find out when the pain occurs. How long does it last? Is it worse in the morning or evening?
• What does the pain feel like? Is it burning, throbbing, aching, or stabbing? What makes the pain better or worse?
• Ask if he has associated symptoms, such as itching or burning eyes, a headache, or visual changes.
• Has he recently experienced trauma or undergone surgery?

Analyzing the chief complaint. Ranging from mild to severe, eye pain can be a burning, throbbing, aching, or stabbing sensation in or around the eyes. It may also feel as

ANATOMY

Reviewing eye structures

These illustrations show the anatomic structures of the eye. Note that the eye shown below is closed.

EYE

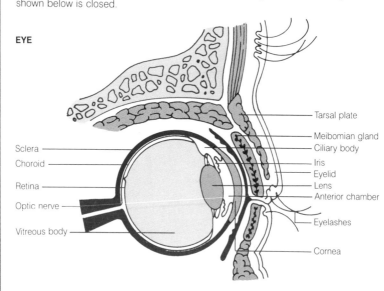

- Tarsal plate
- Meibomian gland
- Ciliary body
- Iris
- Eyelid
- Lens
- Anterior chamber
- Eyelashes
- Cornea

Sclera
Choroid
Retina
Optic nerve
Vitreous body

---

though a foreign body is in the eye.

Eye pain most commonly results from corneal abrasion. But other eye disorders such as glaucoma, trauma such as a chemical burn, and neurologic and systemic disorders can also stimulate the nerve endings in the cornea or external eye, causing pain.

If the eye pain results from a chemical burn, notify the doctor at once. Then irrigate the eye with at least 1 liter of normal saline solution, as hospital policy directs.

Eye discharge. If your patient complains of eye discharge, explore his problem by asking appropriate questions from this list.
- When did the discharge begin?

Does it occur in one or both eyes?
- Does the patient notice the discharge at certain times of the day or in connection with a particular activity? Or is the discharge continuous? Find out if anything makes the discharge better or worse.
- Does he have associated symptoms, such as any pain, burning, itching, or eye tearing? If he has pain, where is it? Have him describe the pain.
- Ask if his eyes are sensitive to light. Does he normally wear glasses or contact lenses?

Analyzing the chief complaint. Usually associated with conjunctivitis, eye discharge refers to the excretion of any substance other than tears.

EYE MUSCLES

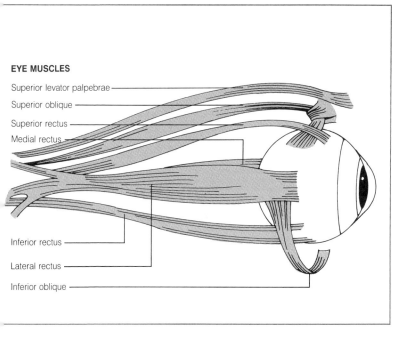

Superior levator palpebrae

Superior oblique

Superior rectus

Medial rectus

Inferior rectus

Lateral rectus

Inferior oblique

You may see slight to copious amounts of discharge from one or both eyes. The discharge may be purulent, frothy, mucoid, cheesy, or ropy. (See *Collecting eye discharge,* page 74.)

Eye discharge commonly results from inflammatory and infectious eye disorders. But certain systemic disorders, such as herpes zoster ophthalmicus and erythema multiforme major (Stevens-Johnson syndrome), can also cause eye discharge. Keep in mind that eye discharge can signal a vision-threatening disorder; your patient may need not only rapid assessment but quick treatment.

Visual changes. If your patient complains of visual changes, explore his problem by asking appropriate questions from this list.
• When did he first notice the visual changes? Did they develop suddenly or gradually? How long have they lasted?
• Ask if the changes affect one or both eyes. Is only a portion of his vision affected? Can he see at all?
• Are the changes constant or intermittent? Do they occur only at certain times?
• Find out if he has associated symptoms, such as eye pain or discharge or a headache.
• Has he recently had eye surgery or has his eye been injured? If so, how soon afterward did he notice the vision changes?

Collecting eye discharge

If your patient has eye discharge, you'll need to collect and examine it. But sometimes, you won't see enough discharge for a specimen. When this happens, you can milk more fluid from the eye by pressing the tear sac, punctum, meibomian gland, or canaliculus lacrimalis.

• When was the last time he had his eyes examined? Does he have hypertension, diabetes, or another medical problem?
• Does he take any medications? What kind? How often does he take them?

Analyzing the chief complaint. Visual changes can range from a loss of visual acuity to total vision loss. The changes can come on suddenly or gradually and can be temporary or permanent. They may result from trauma, certain drugs, or neurologic, ocular, or systemic disorders, including those that cause vascular complications such as diabetes mellitus. Visual blurring, the most common complaint, also can result from mucus passing over the cornea, refractive errors, and improperly fitted contact lenses.

If your patient has visual blurring with a history of trauma; sudden vision loss; sudden, severe eye pain; or a penetrating eye injury, don't touch his eye. Call the doctor at once.

Diplopia. If your patient complains of double vision, explore his problem by asking appropriate questions from this list.
• When did he first notice the dou-

ble vision? Does it affect one or both eyes? Near or far vision? Do the images look as if they're side-by-side, one on top of the other, or both?
• Is the double vision constant or intermittent? Does it get worse at certain times of the day? Does anything make it better or worse?
• Ask if he gets a headache with the double vision.
• Does he normally wear contact lenses?
• Has he recently had eye surgery or have his eyes been injured? If so, how soon afterward did he notice the double vision?
• When was the last time he had his eyes examined?
• Does he take any medications? What kind? How often does he take them?

Analyzing the chief complaint. Diplopia, or double vision, results when the extraocular muscles fail to work together, causing images to fall on noncorresponding parts of the retina. This muscle incoordination can be caused by orbital lesions, surgery, or impaired function of cranial nerves III, IV, and VI (the oculomotor, trochlear, and abducens nerves), which supply the extraocular muscles.

Diplopia usually begins intermittently and affects near or far vision exclusively. Binocular diplopia may result from ocular deviation or displacement, extraocular muscle palsies, or psychoneurosis. This disorder may also follow retinal surgery. Monocular diplopia may result from an early cataract, retinal edema or scarring, a subluxated lens, a poorly fitted contact lens, or an uncorrected refractive error. Diplopia can signal a serious neurologic disorder calling for prompt intervention.

Photophobia. If your patient complains of light sensitivity, explore his problem by asking appropriate questions from this list.
• When did the patient first notice the light sensitivity? Find out how severe it is. Does anything relieve it or make it worse?
• Does he feel any pain? What kind? Where is it?
• Does the patient notice any changes in his vision? If so, what kind?
• Ask if he normally wears contact lenses.
• Has his eye recently been injured or has he had a recent infection?
• Does he take any medications? What kind and how often?

Analyzing the chief complaint. Photophobia often isn't associated with any underlying pathology. The problem may stem from the excessive use of or poorly fitted contact lenses. However, the problem can also result from a systemic disorder such as acute bacterial meningitis or migraines, an ocular disorder such as corneal abrasion, or the use of certain drugs like atropine, amphetamines, or cocaine.

Physical assessment
While performing your physical assessment, keep in mind the basic anatomy of the eyes along with the normal assessment findings. (See *Eyes: Normal findings,* page 76.)
To rapidly assess the eyes, you'll mainly use inspection and palpation.

Inspection. Begin your physical assessment by inspecting the general appearance of your patient's eyes. Stand in front of him and ask him to look at your face. Inspect his eyebrows for symmetrical shape and movement and note the position of his eyeballs.

Appearance. Look for signs of edema, scaling, and lesions on your patient's eyelids, and note if his eye lashes are evenly distributed and curve outward. Ask him to close and open his eyes, making sure the lids close symmetrically and completely. If his eyelids droop at or below the pupil, suspect an oculomotor lesion; if they droop below the middle of the iris, suspect ptosis.
Next, check the position and color of the eyelids, comparing the color with the rest of the face. Look for scaling, lesions, or lumps. If the eyelids have turned outward because of lost elasticity, they'll block tear drainage; if they've turned inward because of spasms or scarring from frequent sties, they may cause corneal irritation and abrasion.
Look at the eyes for nystagmus (involuntary, rapid jerking movements) and lid lag. Note any excessive dryness or tearing.
Next, inspect the bulbar and palpebral conjunctivae, noting any discoloration or opacity (see *Inspecting the conjunctivae,* page 77). Excessive redness and drainage may signal conjunctivitis. Then look at the sclera. Note any color changes, usually a sign of a systemic problem — jaundice from liver disease, for instance, turns the sclera yellow.
Using a penlight and shining it into your patient's eye from several angles, inspect the color, shape, and clarity of the iris. If you can't illuminate a portion of the iris when you shine the penlight into the side of the eye, increased ICP may have changed the depth of the anterior chamber. If you note cloudiness, suspect a cataract.
Also check the shape and clarity of the cornea. If you note inflammation and your patient complains of pain and photophobia, he may have corneal abrasions.

CHECKLIST

Eyes: Normal findings

Inspection
Normal findings include:
- [ ] no edema, scaling, or lesions on eyelids
- [ ] eyelids completely covering the corneas when closed
- [ ] eyelid color the same as surrounding skin color
- [ ] palpebral fissures of equal height
- [ ] margin of upper lid falling between superior pupil margin and superior limbus
- [ ] symmetrical, lesion-free upper eyelids that don't lag or droop when the patient opens his eyes
- [ ] evenly distributed eyelashes that curve outward
- [ ] globe of eye neither protruding from nor sunken into orbit
- [ ] eyebrows with equal size, color, and distribution
- [ ] no nystagmus
- [ ] clear conjunctiva with visible small blood vessels and no signs of drainage
- [ ] white sclera visible through conjunctiva
- [ ] symmetrical irises that are the same color
- [ ] a transparent anterior chamber that contains no visible material when you shine a penlight into the side of the eye
- [ ] transparent, smooth, and bright cornea with no visible irregularities or lesions
- [ ] closing of the lids of both eyes when you stroke each cornea with a wisp of cotton, a test of cranial nerve V (trigeminal nerve)
- [ ] pupils that are equal and round and react normally to light and accommodation
- [ ] lacrimal apparatus free of exudate, swelling, and excessive tearing
- [ ] constriction of both pupils when you shine a light on one
- [ ] proper eye alignment
- [ ] parallel eye movement with each of the six cardinal fields of gaze.

Palpation
Normal findings include:
- [ ] eyelids that don't feel swollen or tender
- [ ] globes that feel equally firm without feeling too hard or spongy
- [ ] lacrimal sacs that don't regurgitate fluid.

Performing tests. Check corneal reflex by lightly stroking a wisp of cotton across the surface of the cornea. Note any asymmetrical responses.

Then check the pupils, using the acronym PERRLA as a guide: Pupils Equal, Round, React to Light, Accommodation. An asymmetrical response or pupillary inequality usually results from a central nervous system disorder or trauma. If you note a change in the contour of the pupil, suspect trauma or iritis. Pupillary constriction may result

from narcotics or pilocarpine; dilation can result from trauma or a systemic reaction to a sympathomimetic or parasympathetic drug.

If your patient has suffered facial or eye trauma or you suspect a neurologic deficit, test extraocular muscle function, using the six cardinal fields of gaze (see *Assessing extraocular muscle function*, page 79).

Palpation. After inspection, gently palpate the eyelids for swelling or tenderness. Eyelid edema without inflammation can signal a poten-

Inspecting the conjunctivae

Inspect the bulbar and palpebral conjunctivae as described below.

Bulbar conjunctiva
• Gently evert your patient's lower eyelid with your thumb or index finger to reveal the inside lower lid.
• Ask her to look up, down, left, and right as you examine her entire lower eyelid.

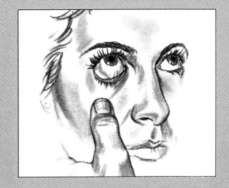

Palpebral conjunctiva
• Ask the patient to look down while you gently pull the medial eyelashes forward and upward with your thumb and index finger to reveal the inside of the upper lid.

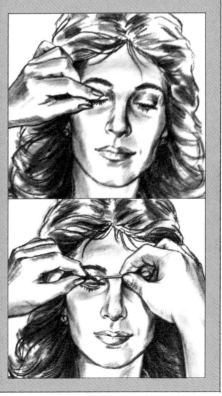

• While holding the eyelashes, press on the tarsal border with a cotton-tipped applicator to evert the eyelid, causing as little discomfort to your patient as possible. Hold the lashes against her eyebrow and examine the conjunctiva, which should look pink and unswollen.
• To invert the eyelid, release the eyelashes and ask your patient to look upward. If that doesn't work, grasp the eyelashes and gently pull them forward.

tially serious condition such as heart disease, glomerulonephritis, or nephrotic syndrome. Then palpate the eyeballs by placing the tips of both index fingers on the eyelids over the sclera while the patient looks down. If you note any hardness, suspect increased intraocular pressure. Next, press your index finger against the patient's lower orbital rim on the side closest to his nose and gently palpate the lacrimal sac. Note any signs of pain, redness, discharge, or excessive tearing.

After obtaining a history and performing a physical assessment, you'll begin to form a diagnostic impression. (See *Eyes: Interpreting your findings,* pages 80 and 81.)

Pediatric considerations
A child may be anxious when anything approaches his eye. So during the examination, try to alleviate his anxiety. Have his parent help by soothing, distracting, or holding him.

When examining an infant, remember that the lacrimal apparatus doesn't develop until age 3 months. When you examine any child, keep in mind that aberrations in eye placement or position may indicate a congenital abnormality.

You'll need to test extraocular muscle function in a child to detect strabismus, a misalignment of the eye's optic axis. *Noncomitant* or *paralytic strabismus* stems from a paralyzed ocular muscle and usually results from eye trauma. You won't detect this type of strabismus when the child looks straight ahead. Instead, you'll note it only when you test the six cardinal fields of gaze. This disorder should resolve 1 to 2 months after the trauma.

A common finding in infants, *concomitant strabismus*—apparent even when the infant looks straight

ahead—should resolve by age 6 months. Some children show signs of strabismus only when they're tired or ill. So ask the parents if they've noticed any unusual eye movements.

Brief periods of nystagmus are normal in an infant who can't yet focus. A child may demonstrate slight nystagmus when gazing to either side. But continuous nystagmus calls for further examination by an ophthalmologist.

Geriatric considerations
Besides affecting the appearance of the eyes, aging causes several changes in perception.

Overall appearance. With aging, the eyebrows and eyelashes thin as the number of hair follicles decreases. You'll also notice that an elderly patient's eyes may appear sunken because of fatty-tissue loss, and dry and lackluster because of decreased tear production. Your patient may complain that his eyes feel dry and that blinking makes them feel gritty. You may also notice lax eyelids, which can lead to eversion or inversion of the lower lids, and pseudoptosis, a drooping of the upper lids caused by aging, not a neurologic problem. On the eyelid, you may see a yellow lipid substance, caused by a thickening of the bulbar conjunctiva on the nasal side.

An elderly patient may have a thin, gray-white ring around the cornea, called arcus senilis. Sclerotic changes over the iris may cloud the cornea and somewhat fixate the pupils, which also look more constricted and react more slowly to light. If the pupils don't react to light at all, however, you should suspect an underlying disorder—unless the patient is over age 85. Only one-third of these patients react to

Assessing extraocular muscle function

If any of the six extraocular muscles or three pairs of cranial nerves (III, IV, and VI) that control eye movement is impaired, your patient will have improper eye alignment, impaired eye movement, and diplopia. Here's how to check for impaired extraocular muscle function.

First, check your patient's corneal light reflex by shining a penlight directly between his eyes, holding it 12″ to 15″ (30.5 to 38.1 cm) away. You'll see a small dot of light at the same spot on each cornea, equidistant from his nose. If the dots are asymmetrical, your patient may have muscle impairment.

Next, check specific muscle and nerve function. Ask your patient to follow your finger (or a pencil) with his eyes as you trace the six cardinal fields of gaze in front of his face (see the illustration). Stop at each field and observe your patient's eyes. If both eyes don't follow your finger into each field of gaze, suspect muscle entrapment or paralysis, with possible nerve damage.

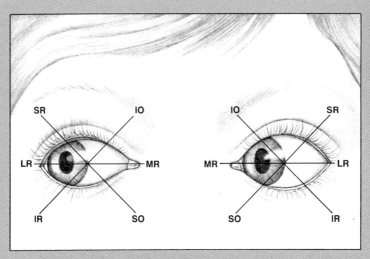

SIX CARDINAL FIELDS OF GAZE	CORRESPONDING MUSCLE
Straight nasal	Medial rectus (MR)
Up and nasal	Inferior oblique (IO)
Down and nasal	Superior oblique (SO)
Straight temporal	Lateral rectus (LR)
Up and temporal	Superior rectus (SR)
Down and temporal	Inferior rectus (IR)

DIAGNOSTIC IMPRESSION

Eyes: Interpreting your findings

After you assess the patient, a group of findings may lead you to suspect a particular disorder. The chart below shows you some common groups of findings for the chief complaints of the eyes, along with the appropriate nursing diagnostic categories and probable causes.

CHIEF COMPLAINT AND FINDINGS	NURSING DIAGNOSTIC CATEGORIES	PROBABLE CAUSE
Eye pain		
• Blurred vision • Decreased visual acuity • Excessive blinking • History of eye trauma or contact lens use • Increased tearing • Irregular corneal surface on inspection	• Pain • Potential for injury • Visual sensory-perceptual alterations	Corneal abrasion
• Sudden onset of severe pain • Conjunctival inflammation • Excessive tearing • Foreign body sensation • Vision intact	• Anxiety • Pain • Self care deficit • Visual sensory-perceptual alterations	Foreign body in the conjunctiva
Eye discharge		
• Purulent drainage • Eye discomfort or pain • Foreign body sensation • Increased tearing • Photophobia • Reddened conjunctivae • Sticky, crusted eyelids	• Potential for infection • Potential for injury • Visual sensory-perceptual alterations	Bacterial conjunctivitis
Visual changes		
• Decreased visual acuity • Perception of halos around lights • Sudden unilateral blurring • Cloudy cornea • Moderately dilated, nonreactive pupil • Severe pain	• Pain • Potential for injury • Visual sensory-perceptual alterations	Acute closed-angle glaucoma
• Sudden appearance of unilateral visual floaters and spots • History of mild hypertension • No history of allergies	• Anxiety • Fear • Knowledge deficit • Potential for injury • Visual sensory-perceptual alterations	Retinal detachment

DIAGNOSTIC IMPRESSION

Eyes: Interpreting your findings *(continued)*

CHIEF COMPLAINT AND FINDINGS	NURSING DIAGNOSTIC CATEGORIES	PROBABLE CAUSE
Diplopia		
• Abnormal pupillary response • Decreased level of consciousness • Emotional lability • Eye deviation • Headache • Hearing loss • Motor weakness • Nystagmus • Paralysis • Seizures • Visual field cuts • Vomiting	• Anxiety • Potential for injury • Self care deficit • Visual sensory-perceptual alterations	Brain tumor
• Recent onset of diplopia • Dilated, unresponsive pupil • Exotropia • History of diabetes mellitus • No eye movement • Ptosis	• Anxiety • Fear • Knowledge deficit • Potential for injury • Visual sensory-perceptual alterations	Extraocular motor nerve palsy
Photophobia		
• Changes in color perception • Gradual blurring and loss of vision • Perception of halos around lights • Visible white area behind pupil on inspection with penlight	• Potential for injury • Visual sensory-perceptual alterations	Cataract
• Conjunctival injection • Eye discomfort • Slightly blurred vision	• Anxiety • Potential for injury • Self care deficit • Visual sensory-perceptual alterations	Posterior uveitis

light, and most show little if any accommodation.

Perception changes. As the lens thickens and yellows with age, a person's light perception diminishes and his color perception becomes distorted. An elderly patient may identify blues and purples as green, for instance. The yellow, more opaque lens also causes glare and cuts down visual acuity in dim light. Distance perception also decreases with age, making it hard for an elderly patient to distinguish objects clearly at a distance.

Usually a normal finding in an elderly patient, decreased peripheral vision may also result from decreased intraocular fluid reabsorption and signal glaucoma. If peripheral vision decreases suddenly and your patient complains of eye pain, suspect acute glaucoma — a medical emergency. Notify the doctor at once.

Ears

When a patient has a complaint related to the ears, such as hearing loss, tinnitus, or ear pain, perform your rapid assessment as described below. (See *Reviewing ear structures.*)

General observations
Begin by making sure both ears are present. Note their shape, contour, and color and look for any obvious lesions, drainage, or swelling.

Then assess your patient's gross hearing ability by whispering or holding a ticking watch by each ear. Look for hearing aids. Next, listen to your patient's tone of voice and note any irregularities such as excessive loudness.

Vital signs
Check the patient's vital signs, particularly his temperature, a key indicator of ear infection. Changes in pulse rate and blood pressure may result from CSF leaking from the ears, a sign of a head injury.

History
After completing your general observations and vital signs check, obtain a quick history of the patient's chief complaint.

For the ears, such complaints include earache, hearing loss, tinnitus, and vertigo. Use these critical questions to gather the essential information.

Earache. If your patient complains of an earache, explore his problem by asking appropriate questions from this list.
• When did he first notice the earache? Did it start suddenly or gradually? How long has he had it?
• Where does it hurt? Does he feel the pain in one or both ears?
• Have the patient describe the pain. Is it constant or intermittent? Does he feel it only when someone touches or pulls on the ear? Does anything make the pain better or worse?
• Determine whether he has any associated symptoms, such as itching or ringing in his ears. Does he feel dizzy? Do his ears feel blocked? Does he have trouble swallowing? What about neck or mouth pain?
• Has he recently had any problems with his eyes, mouth, teeth, jaws, sinuses, or throat? Did he just have a cold? Has he recently been hit on the ear?

Analyzing the chief complaint. Ear pain can range in severity from a feeling of fullness or blockage to deep pain; at times, it may be difficult to localize. The pain may be intermittent or continuous and may develop gradually or suddenly.

Ear pain usually results from disorders of the external and middle ear associated with infection, obstruction (from earwax or a foreign body), or trauma. Less frequently, such pain results from an inner ear infection or is referred from adjacent areas, including the nose, mouth, sinuses, hypopharynx, and temporomandibular joint.

The particular symptoms your patient describes and the signs you observe help pinpoint the cause. Pain caused by touching or pulling the ear, for instance, usually indicates an external ear infection; a

ANATOMY

Reviewing ear structures

This illustration shows the anatomic structures of the ear.

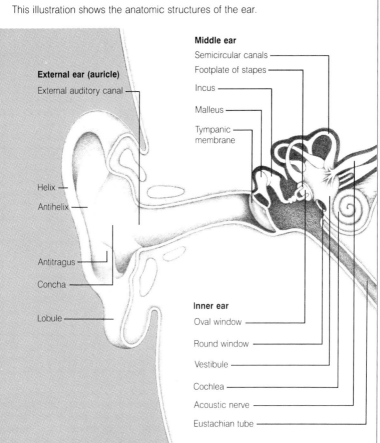

External ear (auricle)
External auditory canal
Helix
Antihelix
Antitragus
Concha
Lobule

Middle ear
Semicircular canals
Footplate of stapes
Incus
Malleus
Tympanic membrane

Inner ear
Oval window
Round window
Vestibule
Cochlea
Acoustic nerve
Eustachian tube

deep, throbbing pain often comes from a middle ear disorder. A severely inflamed outer ear may result from a swollen or completely blocked ear canal. A feeling of pressure or blockage can stem from a eustachian tube dysfunction that creates negative pressure in the middle ear or from muscle spasm or temporomandibular joint arthralgia.

Hearing loss. If your patient complains of a hearing loss, explore his problem by asking appropriate questions from this list.
• When did he first notice a change in his hearing? Did it happen suddenly or gradually? How long has it lasted?
• Is the hearing loss continuous or intermittent? In one ear or both?

Does anything make it better or worse?

• Ask the patient if he sometimes shouts during a conversation or frequently has to ask others to repeat what they said. Does he often turn up the radio or television? Do voices sound muffled?

• Does he have associated symptoms, such as ear pain or ringing, hissing, or other unusual sounds in his ears?

• Does he frequently have ear infections? Has he ever had ear surgery or been hit on the ear? Does anyone else in his family have trouble hearing?

• Find out if he's recently taken any medications, such as antibiotics.

Analyzing the chief complaint. Hearing loss may be temporary or permanent, partial or complete, and may involve reception of low-, middle-, or high-frequency tones. It can be classified as conductive, sensorineural, mixed, or functional.

Conductive hearing loss results from disorders of the external and middle ear that block sound transmission. Sensorineural hearing loss (nerve deafness) results from disorders of the inner ear or cranial nerve VIII (vestibulocochlear nerve). Mixed hearing loss combines aspects of both conductive and sensorineural hearing loss. Functional hearing loss results from psychological factors; no identifiable organic damage exists.

Hearing loss may be caused by trauma, infection, allergy, tumors, certain systemic and hereditary disorders, and certain ototoxic drugs and treatments. The most common type of hearing loss is presbycusis—a sensorineural hearing loss that usually affects those over age 50. Other physiologic causes include ear wax impaction, barotitis media

(resulting from a descent in an airplane or elevator, diving, or being close to an explosion), and chronic exposure to noise over 90 decibels. Such exposure can occur at work, with a hobby, or while listening to music.

Tinnitus. If your patient complains of tinnitus, explore his problem by asking appropriate questions from this list.

• When did the patient first notice the abnormal sound? Does he notice it in one or both ears?

• Have him describe the sound. Is it a ringing or buzzing sound? Does it sound like air escaping? Is it high-pitched or low-pitched? Constant or intermittent?

• Does anything make it better or worse?

• Does he have associated symptoms, such as vertigo, a hearing loss, or headache along with the sound?

Analyzing the chief complaint. Although tinnitus literally means ringing in the ears, several abnormal sounds fall under this term. Your patient may describe the noise as sounding like escaping air, running water, or the inside of a seashell. Or he may describe it as a sizzling, buzzing, or humming noise. Tinnitus can be unilateral or bilateral, constant or intermittent. It's classified according to who hears it—the patient only or both patient and nurse, who listens with a stethoscope—and according to where the patient hears it—in his ears or his head.

Tinnitus results from the stimulation of sensory auditory neurons, which transmit a sound impulse. Commonly resulting from ear disorders, tinnitus may also stem from cardiovascular and systemic disorders. Certain drugs, such as aspirin and aminoglycosides, can also produce tinnitus.

Vertigo. If your patient complains of vertigo, explore his problem by asking appropriate questions from this list.
• When did the patient first notice the vertigo? Did it begin suddenly or gradually? Is it constant or intermittent? How long does an attack last?
• What was he doing before the vertigo started?
• Has he had such attacks before? When? How often do they occur and how long do they last?
• Does it feel as if he's moving or as if the surroundings are moving around him? Can he walk during a vertigo attack or must he sit or lie down? Has he ever fallen because of an attack?
• Find out if anything relieves the vertigo or makes it worse.
• Does he have associated symptoms, such as nausea and vomiting or hearing loss?
• Does he take any medications? What kind? How often does he take them?

Analyzing the chief complaint. Vertigo is an illusion of movement in which the patient feels that he's revolving or that his surroundings are revolving around him. He may also complain of feeling as though he's being pulled sideways, as if drawn by a magnet. Vertigo usually begins abruptly and may be temporary or permanent, mild or severe. It worsens when the patient moves and often subsides when he lies down. A patient may confuse it with dizziness, a sensation of imbalance and light-headedness that doesn't include the whirling sensation. And unlike dizziness, vertigo is often accompanied by nausea, vomiting,

nystagmus, and tinnitus or hearing loss.

Vertigo can result from an underlying physiologic cause, such as a neurologic or otologic disorder that affects the equilibratory apparatus. (This apparatus includes the vestibule, semicircular canals, cranial nerve VIII, vestibular nuclei in the brain stem and their temporal lobe connections, and the eyes.) But vertigo can also stem from alcohol intoxication, hyperventilation, and postural changes, as well as from certain tests, procedures, and drugs, including salicylates and aminoglycosides.

Physical assessment
While performing your physical assessment, keep in mind the basic anatomy of the ears, along with normal assessment findings. (See *Ears: Normal findings,* page 86.) To rapidly assess the ears, you'll mainly use inspection and palpation.

Inspection. Begin by looking at the outer ear, or auricle, noting placement, color, size, and bilateral symmetry. A deviation in the alignment of the auricles suggests renal or chromosomal abnormalities. Pale or excessively red ears may point to an underlying vasomotor disorder; red ears can also signal a fever. Exceptionally large or small or unusually shaped ears may result from an injury or abnormality such as a congenital disorder. Or they may simply be a family trait.

Next, look for drainage, nodules, or lesions. Check behind the ears, too, looking for inflammation, masses, or lesions. Purulent drainage usually results from an infection; clear or bloody drainage may be leaking CSF. Then examine the entrance of the external auditory canal. Observe the color, and note

Ears: Normal findings

Inspection
Normal findings include:
□ bilaterally symmetrical, proportionately sized auricles that have a vertical measurement between 1½" and 4" (4 cm to 10 cm)
□ tip of ear crossing eye-occiput line (an imaginary line extending from the lateral aspect of the eye to the occipital protuberance)
□ long axis of ear perpendicular to (or no more than 10 degrees from perpendicular to) the eye-occiput line
□ ear color that matches color of facial skin
□ no signs of inflammation, lesions, or nodules
□ no cracking, thickening, scaling, or lesions behind the ear when you bend the auricle forward
□ no visible discharge from auditory canal
□ a patent external meatus
□ skin color on the mastoid process that matches the skin color of the surrounding areas
□ no redness or swelling.

Palpation
Normal findings include:
□ no masses or tenderness on the auricle
□ no tenderness on the auricle or tragus during manipulation
□ either small, nonpalpable lymph nodes on the auricle or discrete, mobile lymph nodes with no signs of tenderness
□ well-defined, bony edges on the mastoid process with no signs of tenderness.

any drainage or signs of a foreign body.

Palpation. After inspection, gently palpate the auricles, noting the texture and any tenderness. Also check the elasticity and consistency of the cartilage. Fold the auricle forward to make sure it recoils. Then palpate for swelling, nodules, and lesions you may not have noticed on inspection.

Gently pull the helix backward to assess the external canal. Then pull the auricle and press the tragus. Note any signs of pain, tenderness, or swelling. If your patient has a painful external canal and noticeable yellow, serous, or purulent discharge, or a swollen or sensitive tragus, he may have an infected external or middle ear. A painful tragus accompanied by a swollen external canal and light mucopurulent drainage, for instance, may signal external otitis. If your patient has pain behind the ear over the mastoid area but no pain when you manipulate his auricle, he may have otitis media. This infection may also cause a foul-smelling mucopurulent drainage from the ear, and if it spreads to the labyrinth, vertigo. Then palpate the mastoid process, noting temperature and any tenderness.

After obtaining a history and performing the physical assessment, you'll begin to form a diagnostic impression. (See *Ears: Interpreting your findings.*)

Pediatric considerations
Ask the parent to hold an infant or young child in his lap and immobilize the head with one hand and the arms with the other. Then evaluate the child's gross hearing by observing the way he responds to voices, noises, and the sound of a toy such as a rattle.

As you examine the child, pay close attention to how his auricles are positioned; low-set ears may

DIAGNOSTIC IMPRESSION

Ears: Interpreting your findings

After you assess the patient, a group of findings may lead you to suspect a particular disorder. The chart below shows you some common groups of findings for the chief complaints of the ears, along with the appropriate nursing diagnostic categories and probable causes.

CHIEF COMPLAINT AND FINDINGS	NURSING DIAGNOSTIC CATEGORIES	PROBABLE CAUSE
Earache		
• Pain aggravated by pulling back and up on the auricle or tragus • Feeling of blockage • Foul-smelling, tenacious drainage • History of swimming • Low-grade fever • Swelling of the tragus, external meatus, and external canal	• Auditory sensory-perceptual alterations • Pain • Potential altered body temperature	Acute external otitis
• Severe, throbbing ear pain • Feeling of fullness in ear • Fever • Mild hearing loss • Nausea and vomiting • Slight dizziness	• Auditory sensory-perceptual alterations • Hyperthermia • Knowledge deficit	Acute serous otitis media
Hearing loss		
• Family history of otosclerosis • History of progressive loss • Patient speaks softly despite complaining of hearing loss • Slight dizziness • Tinnitus	• Auditory sensory-perceptual alterations • Potential for injury	Otosclerosis
• Bilateral hearing loss • Dizziness • Feeling of fullness in ear • Itching	• Anxiety • Auditory sensory-perceptual alterations • Potential for infection • Potential for injury	Cerumen impaction
Tinnitus		
• Sudden onset of tinnitus • Feeling of fullness in the ears • Hearing loss • Pain • Vertigo	• Auditory sensory-perceptual alterations • Pain • Potential for injury	Tympanic membrane perforation

(continued)

DIAGNOSTIC IMPRESSION

 Ears: Interpreting your findings *(continued)*

CHIEF COMPLAINT AND FINDINGS	NURSING DIAGNOSTIC CATEGORIES	PROBABLE CAUSE
Tinnitus		
• History of severe arthritis • Mild dizziness • Nausea • Patient taking high doses of salicylates	• Auditory sensory-perceptual alterations • Potential fluid volume deficit • Potential for injury	Salicylate toxicity
Vertigo		
• Sudden onset; attack lasting a few minutes to hours • Low buzzing tinnitus in one ear • Altered ability to perform activities of daily living • Fluctuating low-frequency, sensorineural hearing loss, usually in one ear • Nausea • History of previous episodes; patient is asymptomatic between attacks	• Auditory sensory-perceptual alterations • Potential activity intolerance • Potential for injury • Self care deficit	Meniere's disease
• Gradual onset • Nausea • Spontaneous nystagmus with jerky movement of the eyes toward unaffected ear • Vomiting	• Anxiety • Auditory sensory-perceptual alterations • Hyperthermia	Labyrinthitis

point to one or more birth defects, such as renal agenesis or other anomalies. Other external ear deformities may also signal abnormalities — Down's syndrome, for instance, causes hyperplasia of the superior crus of the antihelix, making the auricle fold over. Keep in mind, too, that the ear canal slants up in a younger child and down in an older child or adult.

Geriatric considerations

As you examine an elderly patient's outer ears, you may notice that the auricle has less fat and harder cartilage than you'd see on a younger adult. Also, the skin and earwax in the external ear canal may be dry and flaky.

Your patient may suffer from a conductive or sensorineural hearing loss — presbycusis, for instance. This sensorineural hearing loss of high-frequency tones eventually results in a loss of all frequencies, making it harder for the patient to hear consonants. Such a hearing loss will make it hard for your patient to understand what you're saying.

Suggested readings

Fuller, J., and Scaller-Ayers, J. *Health Assessment: A Nursing Approach.* Philadelphia: J.B. Lippincott Co., 1990.

Kaufman, J. "Nurse's Guide to Assessing the 12 Cranial Nerves," *Nursing90* 20(6):56-58, June 1990.

Malasanos, L., et al. *Health Assessment,* 4th ed. St. Louis: C.V. Mosby Co., 1989.

Morton, P. *Health Assessment in Nursing.* Springhouse, Pa.: Springhouse Corporation, 1989.

Potter, P. *Pocket Guide to Physical Assessment,* 2nd ed. St. Louis: C.V. Mosby Co., 1990.

Stevens, S., and Becker, K. "A Simple, Step-By-Step Approach to Neurologic Assessment," Part 1. *Nursing88* 18(9):52-61, September 1988.

Stevens, S., and Becker, K. "A Simple, Step-By-Step Approach to Neurologic Assessment," Part 2. *Nursing88* 18(10):51-58, October 1988.

5

ASSESSMENT OF THE CHEST

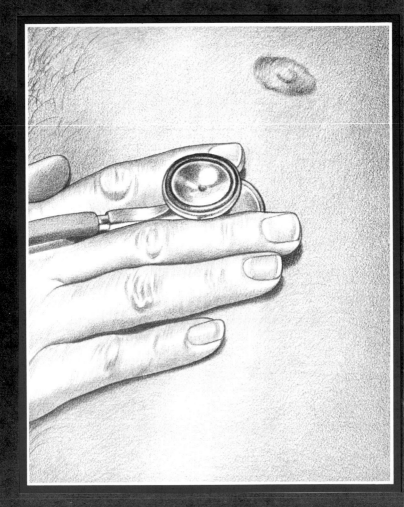

Among the many chest-related problems you're likely to encounter, those affecting the lungs and heart usually pose the gravest threat to the patient. Rapid assessment — and timely intervention — can help you prevent or manage serious complications.

This chapter describes the techniques you'll use to assess the lungs and heart rapidly. Focusing on the most common problems associated with these organs, the chapter provides critical history questions for exploring your patient's chief complaint. Next, you'll find an explanation of how to proceed with the physical examination. Then comes information on interpreting your assessment findings to form an accurate diagnostic impression. The chapter also contains special considerations for pediatric and elderly patients.

Remember that depending on your findings, you may have to interrupt your assessment of the chest to examine another part of the body. Or you may need to stop your assessment to provide emergency intervention.

Lungs

When a patient has a chief complaint related directly to the lungs, you need to focus your rapid assessment accordingly. As time permits, your rapid assessment of the patient's lungs should include general observations, a check of his vital signs, a brief history, and a physical assessment. (See *Reviewing lung structure,* page 92.)

General observations
Observe the patient's level of consciousness (LOC), chest shape and movement, skin condition, and respiratory function.

Level of consciousness. Because the brain needs large amounts of oxygenated blood to function properly, a patient's LOC becomes a sensitive indicator of adequate oxygenation. Alterations in LOC may indicate a problem in the lungs — the organs responsible for oxygenating the blood. Look for signs of change, such as lethargy, agitation, increased anxiety, somnolence, confusion, or irritability.

Chest shape and movement. Examine the patient's chest for overall symmetry, shape, and appearance. With women, observe the position, location, and size of the breasts, noting any deviations. Next, observe the appearance and alignment of the posterior chest and note any deviations in bony structures, such as the scapulae and the thoracic spine. Note any chest deformities that may interfere with expansion (see *Recognizing thoracic deformities,* pages 94 and 95).

Skin condition. Quickly survey the anterior and posterior chest for discoloration or breaks in skin integrity. Observe the skin of the chest area, as well as the extremities and mouth, noting any cyanosis, flushing, or pallor. Look for diaphoresis.

Although both peripheral and central cyanosis are late signs of hypoxia, they stem from different causes. Peripheral cyanosis reflects sluggish peripheral circulation and usually results from a cardiac problem. Central cyanosis reflects excessive amounts of unsaturated hemoglobin in arterial blood, caused by inadequate oxygenation, right-to-left cardiac shunting, or a hemato-

Reviewing lung structure

This illustration shows a cross-sectional view of normal lungs.

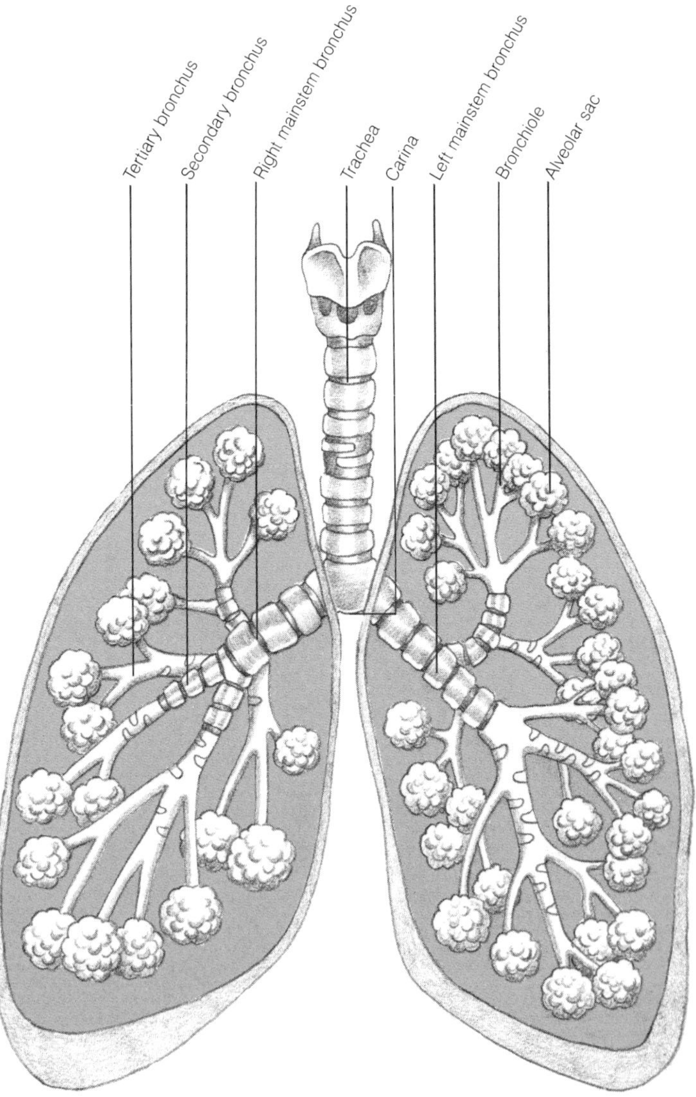

Tertiary bronchus

Secondary bronchus

Right mainstem bronchus

Trachea

Carina

Left mainstem bronchus

Bronchiole

Alveolar sac

logic disorder. You'll find signs of central cyanosis in highly vascular areas, such as the lips, mouth, conjunctivae, and underside of the tongue. With a dark-skinned patient, inspect the areas where cyanotic changes would be most apparent, such as the mucous membranes.

Flushing may indicate increased partial pressures of carbon dioxide in arterial blood, whereas pallor may indicate reduced oxyhemoglobin levels. Diaphoresis may indicate fever, infection, or anxiety, but it can also occur with pulmonary disorders such as pulmonary embolism. Pale, diaphoretic skin may signal early respiratory distress.

Respiratory function. Observe the patient's face for signs of pain, such as grimacing, and signs of respiratory distress, such as nasal flaring. Does he seem short of breath or hoarse when he speaks? Do you hear signs of respiratory distress, such as crowing, wheezing, or stridor? Look at his body position. Is he leaning forward to ease his breathing? Also look for accessory muscle use, and note intercostal and sternal retractions—both signs of serious breathing difficulties.

Check the rate, rhythm, and quality of the patient's respirations. If his respiratory rate is less than 8 breaths/minute, check for other changes in vital signs, a decreased LOC, and pupillary constriction. If the rate is greater than 16 breaths/minute, look for signs of labored breathing. Respirations change in response to hypoxia. Initially, the body will compensate for hypoxia by increasing the respiratory rate and depth. But when the body tires, the rate and depth decrease and respiratory failure may follow.

As you assess the patient's respirations, also note any unusual mouth odor or sputum that may indicate an infection.

Vital signs

Since you've already assessed the patient's respirations, your vital signs check will include only temperature, pulse, and blood pressure. Compare your measurements with his baseline vital signs. Any deviation accompanying a change in his condition may indicate a respiratory problem.

Temperature. Fever commonly indicates respiratory infection, which impairs the diffusion of gases from the lungs to the bloodstream. The metabolic rate rises with temperature, heightening oxygen demand. The combination of impaired diffusion from the infection and a fever above 100.6° F (38.1° C) may make it difficult to meet the body's respiratory needs.

Because of respiratory problems, you may have difficulty obtaining an accurate temperature reading. For instance, an oral temperature may be spuriously low if the patient can't keep his lips closed, if he's receiving humidified oxygen, or if he's tachypneic (respiratory rate greater than 20 breaths/minute). Under these circumstances, consider obtaining a rectal reading.

Pulse. An elevated pulse rate may indicate hypoxia that has developed in response to sympathetic nervous stimulation. Or an elevated rate may stem from pain, fever, exertion, anxiety, or smoking.

An irregular pulse may reflect cardiac arrhythmias, especially in a patient with chronic respiratory problems and hypoxia. An irregular, thready, or weak pulse may also indicate diminished tissue and pulmonary perfusion.

Recognizing thoracic deformities

When you observe your patient's chest, note any deviations from the normal size and shape. In the illustrations below, you'll see a normal adult chest and five

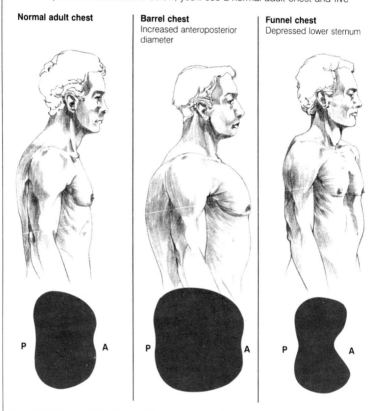

Normal adult chest

Barrel chest
Increased anteroposterior diameter

Funnel chest
Depressed lower sternum

Blood pressure. The patient with a respiratory problem may have normal, elevated, or depressed blood pressure. A change in blood pressure depends on the patient's previous physical condition and his ability to compensate for the existing respiratory difficulty.

With acute respiratory distress, expect blood pressure to be normal initially, or to rise slightly to compensate for the problem. During de-

compensation, blood pressure will fall.

History
During your rapid assessment, obtain a brief history of the patient's chief complaint. Some common lung-related problems include dyspnea, chest pain, coughing, and hemoptysis. Later, when the patient's condition permits, you can obtain a more detailed health history.

chest deformities. The shape below each illustration represents the horizontal cross-sectional view. (A indicates anterior; P indicates posterior.)

Pigeon chest
Anteriorly displaced sternum

Thoracic kyphoscoliosis
Raised shoulder and scapula, thoracic convexity, and flared interspaces

Kyphosis
Rounded thoracic convexity

When taking the history, remember that a patient who suffers from hypoxemia, hypoxia, or hypercapnia may have periods of confusion, inattentiveness, or drowsiness. If this is the case, assess his ability to answer your questions. If necessary, question a family member instead, or postpone your history questions and continue your rapid assessment. If the patient is experiencing shortness of breath, be prepared to ask questions that require a yes-or-no response.

Dyspnea. If your patient complains of dyspnea, explore his problem by asking appropriate questions from this list.
• When did he first become short of breath? How frequent are the attacks?
• Ask the patient if he feels as though he's choking.

ASSESSMENT TIP

How to quantify dyspnea

How your patient characterizes his dyspnea depends on his tolerance for discomfort. What one patient considers to be severe shortness of breath may seem mild to another patient. To make your rapid assessment as objective as possible, ask him to briefly describe how various activities affect his dyspnea. Then document his response using this grading system:

Grade 1
Shortness of breath with mild exertion, such as running a short distance or climbing a flight of stairs

Grade 2
Shortness of breath while walking a short distance at a normal pace on level ground

Grade 3
Shortness of breath with a mild daily activity such as shaving or bathing

Grade 4
Shortness of breath at rest

Grade 5
Shortness of breath when supine

• What was he doing when the attack occurred? What activity level precipitates his dyspnea?
• Does either the patient's position or the time of day affect his breathing?
• Does anything relieve the attacks or make them worse?
• Does he ever wheeze, sweat, cough, or hear a crowing sound when he breathes? Does he have chest pain or feel feverish? Do his lips or nail beds ever turn blue during an attack?
• Does he smoke?

Analyzing the chief complaint. The subjective sensation of difficult or uncomfortable respiration, dyspnea occurs when ventilation is disturbed. When ventilatory demands exceed the actual or perceived capacity of the lungs to respond, the patient becomes short of breath. Decreased lung compliance, a disturbance in the chest bellows system, an airway obstruction, or exogenous factors, such as obesity, can increase the work of breathing.

When you evaluate dyspnea, you face two tasks. First, you must determine whether the patient's dyspnea stems from cardiac or pulmonary disease. Then, you must evaluate the degree of impairment the dyspnea has caused.

Your questions about the onset and severity of your patient's dyspnea should prove helpful. A sudden onset may indicate an acute problem, such as pneumothorax or pulmonary embolus. Sudden dyspnea may also result from anxiety caused by hyperventilation. A gradual onset suggests a slow, progressive disorder, such as emphysema, whereas acute intermittent attacks may indicate asthma.

Precipitating factors also help pinpoint the cause. For instance, dyspnea during sleep (paroxysmal nocturnal dyspnea) or dyspnea when supine (orthopnea) may stem from a chronic lung disorder or a cardiac disorder, such as left ventricular failure. Dyspnea aggravated by activity suggests poor ventilation and perfusion or inefficient breathing mechanisms. (See *How to quantify dyspnea.*)

Chest pain. If your patient complains of chest pain, explore his problem by asking appropriate questions from this list.
• When did he first notice the chest

pain? Is the pain sharp and stabbing, or steady and dull?
• Find out where the pain is located. Does it radiate? Can he point to the painful areas?
• Is the pain constant or intermittent? Ask if some specific activity causes the pain and if anything aggravates it or relieves it.
• Is he breathing normally or deeply when pain strikes? Is it accompanied by other signs and symptoms, such as a cough, difficulty breathing, coughing up of blood, or nausea?

Analyzing the chief complaint. When a patient complains of chest pain, determine first if he has a life-threatening problem. Most structures within or adjacent to the thorax can produce pain, but not all pain indicates a life-threatening problem. Taking a careful history will help you determine the cause of the pain.

If the patient says his pain increases with deep breaths, abates when he sits up, or gets worse with chest-wall movement, his pain probably has a pulmonary origin. The lungs themselves have no pain-sensitive nerve endings, but the thoracic muscles, parietal pleura, and tracheobronchial tree do. The sudden onset of pleuritic pain, accompanied by dyspnea, may indicate pneumothorax or pulmonary embolism — conditions requiring immediate intervention.

Of course, chest pain often signals a cardiac disorder.

Coughing. If your patient complains of a cough, explore his problem by asking appropriate questions from this list.
• How long has he had the cough? Is the cough dry and hacking or productive? If it's productive, have him

Understanding a cough

Coughing protects the lungs by removing mucus and foreign particles from the air passages. A person coughs when something irritates nerve endings somewhere in his respiratory tract — the larynx, trachea, or bronchi. Pleural stimulation can also elicit coughing.

When a cough occurs, first the throat closes and then the diaphragm, abdominal muscles, and chest muscles tighten involuntarily. This increases air pressure in the bronchi and trachea. Then, when the throat suddenly opens, air rushes from the lungs into the trachea, pushing mucus toward the pharynx in an explosive burst.

describe the color and odor of the mucus. How much mucus does he cough up? Does the cough seem worse at a certain time of the day?
• Does he have any breathing difficulties? What about other symptoms?
• Does he smoke?
• Is he taking any medications, such as a cough suppressant?

Analyzing the chief complaint. An important pulmonary defense mechanism, coughing usually indicates a respiratory disorder. (See *Understanding a cough.*) Your task — evaluating the cough — isn't easy because the cause can range from trivial to life-threatening. It may be relatively harmless, such as postnasal drip. Or the cough may stem from asthma or lung cancer.

A severe cough can disrupt daily activities and cause chest pain or acute respiratory distress. An early morning cough may indicate chronic airway inflammation, possibly from cigarette smoke. A late afternoon cough may indicate exposure to irritants. And an evening cough may suggest chronic postnasal drip or sinusitis. A dry cough may signal a cardiac condition; a hacking cough may indicate pneumonia; and a congested cough may indicate a cold, pneumonia, or bronchitis.

Increasing amounts of mucoid sputum may suggest acute tracheobronchitis or acute asthma. If the patient has chronic productive coughs with mucoid sputum, suspect asthma or chronic bronchitis. If the sputum changes from white to yellow or green, suspect a bacterial infection.

Hemoptysis. If your patient complains of hemoptysis, explore his problem by asking appropriate questions from this list.
• How long has he been coughing up blood? How much has he coughed up?
• Have him describe the sputum's color. Is it dark red, blood tinged, or pink and frothy?
• Does he have any other symptoms, such as difficulty breathing?
• Is he taking an anticoagulant?

Analyzing the chief complaint. Coughing up blood-tinged or grossly bloody sputum, hemoptysis has several pathologic causes — including inflammation of the tracheobronchial mucosa, injury to the pulmonary vasculature, and marked elevation in pulmonary capillary pressure. This chief complaint may result from violent coughing or from a serious disorder such as pneumonia, lung cancer, lung abscess, tuberculosis, pulmonary embolism, bronchiectasis, or a cardiac condition such as left ventricular failure. Because of its frightening appearance and serious causes, hemoptysis often alarms patients.

Physical assessment
Most often, you'll use inspection and auscultation to rapidly assess the lungs. You'll find auscultation gives you the most information when examining the chest. Use palpation and percussion if you have time, or if you suspect a condition that these techniques would quickly reveal. For instance, if you suspect pneumothorax, percuss the area over the lungs for hyperresonance to confirm your suspicion.

While performing your assessment, keep in mind the basic anatomy of the lungs and the normal assessment findings. (See *Lungs: Normal findings.*)

Begin by placing the patient in a position that provides access to his posterior and anterior chest. If his condition permits, have him sit on the edge of a bed or examining table or on a chair, leaning forward slightly with his arms folded across his chest. If this isn't possible, place him in the semi-Fowler's position for the anterior chest examination. Then ask him to lean forward slightly and use the side rails or mattress for support while you quickly examine his posterior chest. If he can't lean forward, place him in a lateral position or ask another staff member to help him sit up.

Your physical assessment should cover three areas of the chest: posterior, anterior, and lateral. Where you begin isn't as important as how you proceed. Work systematically, comparing one side of the chest with the other. Be sure to examine the lung apices during the posterior and the anterior examinations.

Inspection. First, inspect the patient's chest for obvious problems, such as draining, open wounds, bruises, abrasions, scars, and cuts. Also look for less obvious problems,

Lungs: Normal findings

Inspection
Normal findings include:
☐ side-to-side symmetrical chest configuration.
☐ anteroposterior diameter less than the transverse diameter, with a 1:2 to 5:7 ratio in an adult.
☐ normal chest shape, with no deformities, such as a barrel chest, kyphosis, retraction, sternal protrusion, or depressed sternum.
☐ costal angle less than 90 degrees, with the ribs joining the spine at a 45-degree angle.
☐ quiet, unlabored respirations with no use of accessory neck, shoulder, or abdominal muscles. You should also see no intercostal, substernal, or supraclavicular retractions.
☐ symmetrically expanding chest wall during respiration.
☐ normal adult respiratory rate, 16 to 20 breaths/minute. Expect some variation depending on the age of your patient.
☐ regular respiratory rhythm, with expiration taking about twice as long as inspiration. Men and children breathe diaphragmatically, while women breathe thoracically.
☐ skin color that matches the rest of the body's complexion.

Auscultation
Normal findings include:
☐ loud, high-pitched bronchial breath sounds over the trachea.
☐ intense, medium-pitched bronchovesicular breath sounds over the mainstem bronchi, between the scapulae, and below the clavicles.
☐ soft, breezy, low-pitched vesicular breath sounds over most of the peripheral lung fields.

Palpation
Normal findings include:
☐ warm, dry skin.
☐ no tender spots or bulges in the chest.

Percussion
Normal findings include:
☐ resonant percussion sounds over the lungs.

ch as rib deformities, fractures, ions, or masses.

Examine the shape of his chest ll. Observe the anteroposterior P) and transverse diameters. If e AP diameter is as large as (or nost as large as) the transverse ameter, suspect emphysema.

Note the patient's respiratory patrn. A prolonged expiratory phase ay indicate an obstructive pulmory disease, such as asthma or emysema. With prolonged expira-ns, you may also note labored, rsed-lip breathing. An irregular spiratory pattern, such as Cheyne-okes respirations, will usually be associated with a central nervous system or metabolic disorder and requires immediate intervention. (See *Assessing respiratory patterns,* page 100.)

Observe the patient's chest movement during respirations. The chest should move upward and outward symmetrically on inspiration. Consider the factors that may affect movement such as pain, poor positioning, or abdominal distention. You may find paradoxical movement of the chest wall if the patient has fractured ribs or flail chest. Or, if one side of the chest doesn't expand as much as the other, the patient

Assessing respiratory patterns

Your patient's respiratory pattern provides important clues to his respiratory status and overall condition. Use the chart below to help identify his pattern.

TYPE	CHARACTERISTICS
Eupnea (normal)	Normal rate and rhythm: adults and teenagers, 12 to 20 breaths/minute; children ages 2 to 12, 20 to 30 breaths/minute; infants, 30 to 50 breaths/minute. Occasional deep breaths (2 to 3 breaths/minute).
Tachypnea	Increased regular respirations (above 20 breaths/minute in adults). If occurring with fever, rate increases about 4 breaths/minute for each degree Fahrenheit above normal.
Bradypnea	Decreased regular respirations (below 10 breaths/minute in adults).
Hyperpnea	Deeper-than-normal respirations at a normal rate.
Apnea	Absent respirations; may be periodic.
Biot's respirations	Faster and deeper than normal respirations with abrupt pauses; breaths of equal depth.
Cheyne-Stokes respirations	Faster and deeper than normal respirations, followed by slower respirations, over a 30- to 170-second period. Alternates with periods of apnea lasting 20 to 60 seconds.
Kussmaul's respirations	Faster and deeper than normal respirations without pauses; over 20 breaths/minute in adults. Breathing sounds labored with deep breaths that resemble sighs.

may have atelectasis or an underlying pulmonary disease.

Check for accessory muscle use and retraction of intercostal spaces during inspiration. Both of these signs may indicate respiratory distress. Sudden, violent intercostal retraction may indicate airway obstruction or tension pneumothorax. Retraction of abdominal muscles during expiration occurs when the body forces air from the alveoli, as in chronic obstructive pulmonary disease (COPD) and other obstructive disorders. Inspiratory intercostal bulging can occur with cardiac enlargement and aneurysms; localized expiratory bulging occurs with rib fractures and flail chest.

Auscultation. The next step in you physical assessment, auscultating breath sounds, helps you detect al normal fluid or mucus accumulatic as well as obstructed air passages

To auscultate the lungs, place th diaphragm of the stethoscope ove all lung fields, posteriorly, anteriorly, and laterally — if time allows. (See *Sequence for auscultation.*) Auscultate the lungs for normal, a normal, adventitious, and absent breath sounds. Classify breath sounds according to their location intensity, characteristics, pitch, a duration during the inspiratory and expiratory phases.

Abnormal breath sounds. Remember that solid tissue transmits sound better than air or fluid, so over an area of consolidation, breath sounds (as well as spoken or whispered sounds) will be louder than normal. However, if pus, fluid, or air is in the pleural space, breath sounds will be quieter than normal. If a foreign body or secretions obstruct a bronchus, breath sounds will be diminished or absent over distal lung tissue. Diminished breath sounds may indicate an obstructed airway, partial or total lung collapse, thickening of the pleurae, emphysema, or chronic lung disease.

Adventitious breath sounds. These sounds, including crackles, gurgles, wheezes, and pleural friction rubs, indicate abnormalities that interfere with oxygen and carbon dioxide exchange. Usually, a patient with an adventitious breath sound has some form of pulmonary disease.

Crackles result from air moving through airways that contain fluid. Heard during both inspiration and expiration, crackles are discrete sounds that vary in pitch and intensity. They're classified as fine, medium, or coarse.

Fine crackles, often called end-inspiratory crackles, are high-pitched sounds heard near the end of inspiration. You'll commonly detect them first in the lung bases. To simulate this sound, hold several strands of hair close to your ear and roll them between your fingers. Fine crackles result from fluid in small airways or small atelectatic areas that expand when the patient breathes deeply. You may hear fine crackles in a patient who has either congestive heart failure (CHF) or pneumonia.

Sequence for auscultation

When auscultating the posterior, anterior, and then the lateral chest, use a sequence that progresses from side to side, as illustrated below. Compare the area on one side of the patient's chest with the corresponding area on the other side.

Posterior sequence

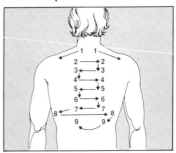

Anterior sequence

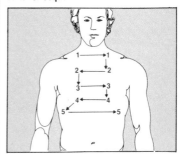

Lateral sequence

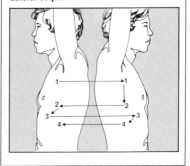

Usually, fine crackles won't clear when the patient breathes deeply or coughs.

Medium crackles result from fluid in slightly larger airways, such as the bronchioles. Lower pitched and coarser than fine crackles, medium crackles occur during the middle or end of inspiration. (Those heard during the middle phase of inspiration are called mid-inspiratory crackles.) Medium crackles won't clear when the patient breathes deeply or coughs.

Coarse crackles result from a large amount of fluid or exudate in the larger upper airways — including the mainstem bronchi and the large bronchi. You'll hear the characteristic loud, bubbling, gurgling sound on both inspiration and expiration. Coarse crackles indicate increasing pulmonary congestion and usually won't clear with deep breathing or coughing.

Gurgles develop when thick secretions partially obstruct airflow through the large upper airways. Loud, coarse, and low-pitched, they resemble snoring. You'll hear gurgles most often on expiration and sometimes on inspiration. A patient may be able to clear gurgles by coughing up secretions.

Wheezes, like gurgles, occur on expiration and sometimes on inspiration. Continuous, high-pitched, musical squeaks, wheezes result when air moves rapidly through airways narrowed by asthma or infection — or when an airway is partially obstructed by a tumor or foreign body. In a patient with mild asthma, you'll probably hear bilateral wheezes on expiration. If his condition worsens, you'll hear wheezes on both expiration and inspiration. Unilateral, isolated wheezes usually indicate a tumor or foreign body obstruction.

Pleural friction rubs have a distinctive grating sound that resembles the sound made by rubbing leather. As the name indicates, these breath sounds result when inflamed visceral and parietal pleurae rub together.

Absent breath sounds. Generally, absent breath sounds are a significant indicator of loss of ventilating power. Underlying causes may include laryngeal bronchospasm, pneumonectomy, phrenic nerve palsy, pneumothorax, hemothorax, or a malpositioned endotracheal tube.

Palpation. Although not routinely part of a rapid assessment, palpation is sometimes indicated. For example, if the patient complains of chest pain, you'll need to palpate his anterior chest using the same sequence you used to auscultate the anterior chest.

Remember, palpation will increase pain in certain disorders, including musculoskeletal pain, irritation of the nerves covering the xiphoid process, or an inflammation of the cartilage connecting the ribs to the sternum (costochondritis). On the other hand, palpation won't increase pain caused by cardiac or pulmonary disorders, such as angina or pleurisy.

Tactile fremitus. If your initial findings indicate that the patient may have tactile fremitus, follow these steps:
• Place your open palm flat against the upper portion of the patient's anterior chest, making sure your fingers don't touch his chest.
• As he repeats a resonant phrase, such as "99, 99," move your hands over his chest from the central airways to the lung periphery, and

back. Systematically move from the top of the suprascapular area to the interscapular area, the infrascapular area, and the hypochondriac area (found at the level of the 5th and 10th intercostal spaces to the right and left of midline). You may have to displace a woman's breasts to examine her anterior chest.

• Repeat this procedure on the posterior chest.

You should feel equally intense vibrations on corresponding sides of the chest. The intensity will vary according to the thickness and structure of the chest, as well as the intensity and pitch of the patient's voice. Note the symmetry of the vibrations and the areas of increased, decreased, or absent fremitus.

Fremitus will be most pronounced in areas of increased airflow, such as the upper chest where the trachea branches into the right and the left mainstem bronchi. You'll feel fremitus most strongly at the second intercostal space on either side of the sternum. Increased fremitus also occurs in areas of lung consolidation, as in pneumonia or atelectasis.

You'll find decreased or absent fremitus over the precordium, over the lung bases, and in areas of decreased airflow. You can also expect to find decreased fremitus with such conditions as emphysema, obesity, pleural effusion, hemothorax, pneumothorax, and pulmonary fibrosis.

Fremitus that occurs at different levels in each lung may indicate a change in the patient's condition, or the development of a new problem.

Percussion. Although not usually performed in a rapid assessment, percussion may be necessary if you suspect a pneumothorax, atelectasis, pleural effusion, or pneumonia. In these cases, use indirect percussion, following the auscultatory sequence described above.

Compare sound variations from one side of the thorax with the other. While you should hear a resonant sound over the lung areas, a dull sound may reflect fluid or solid tissue — indicating pneumonia, atelectasis, or tumors. A flat sound in the lung reflects solid tissue and may indicate atelectasis; a flat sound at the lung bases may indicate pleural effusion. Hyperresonance may reflect air trapped in the lungs, possibly indicating COPD or pneumothorax.

Further assessment. You may need to assess another part of the body to confirm your findings or help identify the underlying cause of a problem. For instance, you may need to assess the patient's heart to determine if his chief complaint is pulmonary- or cardiac-related. You also may need to assess the following:

• the neck for tracheal deviation and jugular vein distention
• the mucous membranes of the mouth and the lips for cyanosis
• the nails beds for cyanosis
• the fingers for clubbing — a sign of chronic respiratory dysfunction.

After obtaining the patient's history and performing a physical assessment, you'll begin to form a diagnostic impression (see *Lungs: Interpreting your findings,* pages 104 and 105).

Pediatric considerations

When you examine infants or young children, keep in mind their stage of growth and development. Alter your assessment techniques accordingly.

Inspection. Before inspecting an infant's chest, first examine his skin. Infants have a thin layer of subcutaneous tissue, making cyanosis a more reliable sign of respiratory

DIAGNOSTIC IMPRESSION

Lungs: Interpreting your findings

After you assess the patient, a group of findings may lead you to suspect a particular disorder. The chart below shows you some common groups of findings for the chief complaints of the lungs, along with the appropriate nursing diagnostic categories and probable causes.

CHIEF COMPLAINT AND FINDINGS	NURSING DIAGNOSTIC CATEGORIES	PROBABLE CAUSE
Dyspnea		
• Accessory muscle hypertrophy • Anorexia • Barrel chest • Chronic productive cough • Diminished breath sounds • History of smoking • Peripheral cyanosis • Prolonged expiration • Pursed-lip breathing • Tachypnea • Weight loss	• Fear (of breathlessness) • Impaired gas exchange • Impaired physical mobility • Ineffective breathing pattern • Pain • Potential for infection • Sleep pattern disturbance	Emphysema
• Dyspnea develops slowly and becomes progressively worse • Decreased breath sounds • Dry cough • Dullness upon percussion • Pleuritic pain that worsens with coughing or deep breathing • Tachycardia • Weight loss	• Altered cardiopulmonary tissue perfusion • Anxiety • Impaired gas exchange • Ineffective airway clearance	Pleural effusion
Unilateral chest pain		
• Pain increases with chest movement; described as sudden, sharp, or severe • Accessory muscle use • Asymmetrical chest expansion • Crepitus • Decreased or absent breath sounds on affected side • Decreased vocal fremitus • Hyperresonance or tympany on affected side • Moderate dyspnea • Nonproductive cough • Restlessness • Tachycardia	• Fear (of chest pain) • Impaired gas exchange • Ineffective breathing pattern • Pain • Sleep pattern disturbance	Pneumothorax

DIAGNOSTIC IMPRESSION

Lungs: Interpreting your findings *(continued)*

CHIEF COMPLAINT AND FINDINGS	NURSING DIAGNOSTIC CATEGORIES	PROBABLE CAUSE
Diffuse chest pain		
• Cyanosis • Diaphoresis • Dry cough • Flaring nostrils • Flushing • Mild wheezing, rhonchi, crackles • Productive cough, audible wheezing, and severe dyspnea develop • Retractions	• Altered cardiopulmonary tissue perfusion • Anxiety • Impaired gas exchange • Ineffective airway clearance • Pain	Asthma
Cough		
• Dyspnea on exertion • Fever • Inspiratory crackles • Mucoid, purulent sputum • Percussion of dull or flat sounds over consolidated area • Pleuritic chest pain • Tachycardia • Tachypnea	• Impaired gas exchange • Ineffective breathing pattern • Pain • Sleep pattern disturbance	Pneumonia
• Fatigue • Headache • Malaise • Mucoid, purulent sputum • Myalgia • Nasal congestion • Rhinorrhea • Sneezing • Sore throat	• Fatigue • Potential ineffective airway clearance	Common cold

distress than it is for adults.

The infant's thorax is rounded, with the AP diameter equal to the transverse diameter. The lateral diameter increases rapidly with growth, so by age 6 the child's proportions will be the same as those of an adult.

Infants and children seldom exhibit hypertrophy of the accessory muscles of respiration. However, they may exhibit bulging or retractions during inspiration and expiration—a sign of breathing difficulty. The intercostal muscles often bulge during infant respiratory distress, while the suprasternal, substernal, and abdominal muscles retract.

Auscultation. Because other assessment procedures may make the child cry, auscultate his lungs right after inspection. Crying increases the respiratory rate and creates noise that interferes with clear auscultation. Because a child's chest is

Sequence for pediatric auscultation

Because an infant or child has a smaller chest than an adult, you need to alter the sequence you use for auscultation. Follow the sequences illustrated below when auscultating the posterior and anterior chest of a pediatric patient.

Posterior sequence

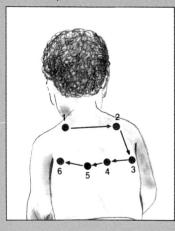

Anterior sequence

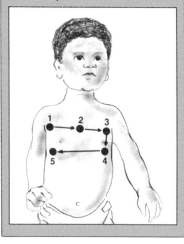

smaller than an adult's, you'll have to adjust your auscultation sequence (see *Sequence for pediatric auscultation*).

Normal pediatric breath sounds are usually louder and harsher than those heard in an adult. Infants and young children may exhibit bronchovesicular sounds throughout the chest, as well as undifferentiated vesicular sounds.

Grunting (deep, low-pitched sounds at the end of each breath) and stridor (loud, harsh, musical sounds) also may be heard — sometimes without even using a stethoscope.

Palpation. Because an infant or a toddler has a small chest, you'll assess only the suprasternal notch. Chest palpation becomes appropriate around age 5.

Percussion. In pediatric patients, percussion usually proves unreliable because of the disproportionate sizes of an infant's chest and an adult's fingers.

Geriatric considerations
While your rapid assessment of an elderly patient will be the same as that for any adult, your findings may differ. For example, the thoracic structure typically becomes rounder with age, and the AP chest diameter increases in relation to the transverse diameter. This results from changes in the thoracic and lumbar spine. The elderly patient may also use accessory muscles to breathe because of calcification of his rib articulations.

Auscultation. When auscultating an elderly patient with suspected atelectasis, begin at the lung bases rather than at the apices. Atelectatic crackles may disappear as the patient repeatedly takes deep breaths. A decreased cough reflex increases the risk of aspiration for this age-group.

Percussion. Never perform blunt percussion on the chest of an elderly woman; osteoporosis may have left her bones brittle. When percussing an elderly patient, you may find hyperresonant sounds that reflect decreased distensibility of the lung tissue.

Heart

When your patient's chief complaint is related directly to the heart, you'll need to focus your rapid assessment accordingly. As with the lungs, rapid assessment of a patient's heart includes general observations, a check of his vital signs, a brief history, and a physical examination. (See *Reviewing heart structure,* page 108.)

If your patient shows signs of a cardiac crisis at any point during the assessment, be prepared to begin emergency procedures immediately.

General observations

Your general observations will provide the first clue of a possible change in your patient's cardiac condition. Observe his LOC, skin condition, and posture and facial expression.

Level of consciousness. Reduced cardiac output can diminish the brain's blood flow and oxygen supply, thereby altering the patient's LOC. Be alert for signs of restlessness, agitation, and irritability. If inadequate brain oxygenation continues,

the patient's LOC will deteriorate from lethargy to disorientation to confusion, and finally, to unresponsiveness.

Skin condition. Look for any changes in the patient's skin color, such as pallor or cyanosis. Pallor occurs when decreased cardiac output or increased sympathetic nervous system activity causes blood vessels to vasoconstrict, shunting blood from the skin to the heart and brain. Sympathetic vasoconstriction also causes peripheral cyanosis—seen in the nail beds, earlobes, and nose. Don't consider cyanosis alone a reliable sign of decreased oxygenation; also feel the patient's arm for warmth and dryness. If his skin feels cool or clammy, suspect peripheral vasoconstriction—possibly an early compensatory response in shock.

When assessing his skin, also look for signs of edema caused by abnormal fluid accumulation in the interstitial spaces.

Posture and facial expression. Assess the patient's posture for signs of discomfort, anxiety, or labored breathing. Observe his facial expression for signs of discomfort, withdrawal, fear, or depression. Expressions of severe anxiety or impending doom should alert you to the seriousness of his situation.

Vital signs

Check the patient's temperature, pulse, respirations, and blood pressure and compare them with his baseline vital signs. Note any deviations.

Temperature. Take the patient's temperature as soon as time allows. An elevated temperature may indicate a cardiovascular inflammation

Reviewing heart structure

This illustration shows a cross-sectional view of a normal heart.

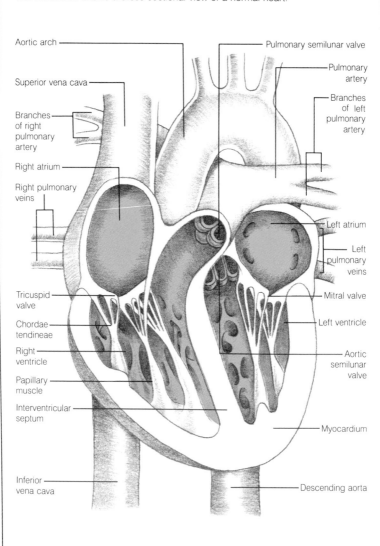

Aortic arch

Superior vena cava

Branches of right pulmonary artery

Right atrium

Right pulmonary veins

Tricuspid valve

Chordae tendineae

Right ventricle

Papillary muscle

Interventricular septum

Inferior vena cava

Pulmonary semilunar valve

Pulmonary artery

Branches of left pulmonary artery

Left atrium

Left pulmonary veins

Mitral valve

Left ventricle

Aortic semilunar valve

Myocardium

Descending aorta

or infection. A mild-to-moderate elevation usually occurs 2 to 5 days after a myocardial infarction (MI), as the healing infarct passes through the inflammatory stage. Acute pericarditis also may cause a similar temperature elevation. Infections, such as subacute bacterial endocarditis, cause fever spikes.

Whatever the cause, an elevated temperature always occurs with increased metabolism, which increases the cardiac work load. Thus, you must watch feverish patients with known heart disease for other signs of increased cardiac work load — such as an increased heart rate.

Pulse. Determine your patient's heart rate by assessing his radial pulse. Quickly palpating the radial pulse for 10 to 15 seconds helps you recognize any gross abnormalities in its rate or rhythm. As soon as possible, palpate the pulse for a minute to detect any problems in rate or quality — especially if you suspect or know he has cardiac disease.

A weak pulse indicates either low cardiac output or increased peripheral vascular resistance, as in arterial atherosclerotic disease. A strong, bounding pulse results from hypertension and high cardiac output states, such as exercise, pregnancy, anemia, and thyrotoxicosis. An irregular pulse or a slow or rapid pulse may indicate an arrhythmia.

Respirations. Count your patient's respirations to determine his breathing pattern. Normally, you'll find eupnea — a regular, unlabored, and bilaterally equal breathing pattern. Tachypnea may indicate a low cardiac output. Dyspnea may indicate CHF but isn't always evident at rest. Listen to the patient speak and note if he must pause every few words to take a breath. A Cheyne-Stokes respiratory pattern may accompany severe heart failure, although it's more commonly associated with coma.

Blood pressure. To accurately measure a patient's blood pressure, first palpate the brachial artery, then auscultate.

Keep in mind that either hypertension or emotional stress associated with the physical assessment may elevate a patient's blood pressure. If you detect an elevated blood pressure, allow the patient to rest for 5 to 10 minutes and then repeat the measurement. This helps determine if the elevation is stress-related or is actually hypertension. The American Heart Association defines hypertension as blood pressure above 140/90 mm Hg on three consecutive readings. Never draw a conclusion from a single reading.

When you assess a patient's blood pressure for the first time, take measurements in both arms. A difference of 10 mm Hg or more between the arms may indicate thoracic outlet syndrome — compression of the arterial flow to one arm produced by pressure from the clavicle or first rib — or another form of arterial obstruction.

After measuring blood pressure, quickly calculate the pulse pressure by determining the difference between the systolic and diastolic pressures. The pulse pressure, which reflects arterial pressure during the resting phase of the cardiac cycle, normally ranges between 30 and 50 mm Hg.

The pulse pressure increases when the stroke volume (output of each ventricle at every contraction) increases, as in exercise, anxiety, or bradycardia (a heart rate of less than 60 beats/minute). Pulse pressure also increases when the peripheral vascular resistance or aortic distensibility decreases, as in anemia, hyperthyroidism, fever, hypertension, aortic coarctation, or aging.

The pulse pressure decreases when a mechanical obstruction exists, such as mitral or aortic stenosis; when the peripheral vessels constrict, as in shock; or when the stroke volume decreases, as in heart failure, hypovolemia, or tachycardia.

History
When time and the patient's condition permit, assess his chief complaint by taking a brief history. Common chief complaints related to the heart include chest pain, dyspnea, palpitations, fatigue, and edema.

Chest pain. If your patient complains of chest pain, explore his problem by asking appropriate questions from this list.
• When did he first notice the pain? What was he doing when it started?
• Find out where the pain is located. Does it radiate? Can he point to the painful areas?
• What type of pain is it? Constant? Intermittent? Have him describe it.
• Does anything aggravate or relieve the pain?
• Does he have any other symptoms he can associate with the pain, such as shortness of breath or an irregular heartbeat?

Analyzing the chief complaint. Sudden, severe chest pain requires prompt evaluation and treatment since it may signal a life-threatening disorder, such as MI. The location and characteristics of the pain, as well as the associated symptoms, help you identify its origin and intervene appropriately.

Although chest pain is one of the most common symptoms of heart disease, it doesn't always originate in the heart. Chest pain can also result from pulmonary and gastroesophageal disorders. (See *Causes of chest pain,* pages 112 and 113.)

Also, cardiac-related pain doesn't always occur in the chest. Pain originating in the heart is transmitted through the thoracic region by the upper five thoracic spinal cord segments. Thus, it may be referred to areas served by the cervical or lower thoracic segments, such as the neck and arms. Upper thoracic segments innervate skin as well as skeletal muscles, making the true origin of the pain hard to determine.

Dyspnea. If your patient complains of dyspnea, explore his problem by asking questions from this list.
• When did he first become short of breath? How frequent are the attacks?
• Find out what activity level triggers the problem. Does his position or the time of day affect his breathing?
• What relieves his attacks? What makes them worse?
• Is his shortness of breath accompanied by cough or any other signs? For instance, do his lips and nail beds turn blue during an attack?
• Does he smoke?

Analyzing the chief complaint. Patients usually report dyspnea as shortness of breath. The degree of patient discomfort caused by dyspnea varies greatly and is often unrelated to the severity of the underlying cause.

Consider dyspnea that occurs at rest or with slight activity as abnormal. When dyspnea occurs gradually over weeks and months, it usually suggests a chronic cardiac problem such as CHF. As the degree of heart failure increases in CHF, lung congestion occurs, leading to dyspnea and coughing. Two types of dyspnea may accompany CHF: orthopnea, which occurs when the patient lies flat; and paroxysmal nocturnal dyspnea, which interrupts sleep and commonly disappears when he sits upright. Orthopnea and paroxysmal nocturnal dyspnea usually result from interstitial pulmonary edema secondary to left ventricular failure.

Sudden dyspnea, accompanied by crushing substernal chest pain that may radiate to the back, neck, jaw, and arms, often indicates MI. In cardiac arrhythmias, dyspnea results from decreased cardiac output and can be acute or gradual. In addition, the pulse rate may be rapid, slow, or irregular, with frequent premature or escape beats.

Dyspnea may also result from coronary artery disease (CAD) and myocardial ischemia, as well as pulmonary disorders, as discussed earlier in the chapter.

Palpitations. If your patient complains of palpitations, explore his problem by asking appropriate questions from this list.
• When did he first notice the palpitations?
• Ask what the sensation feels like. Where does he feel it? How frequently do the attacks occur?
• How long has he been experiencing palpitations? What was he doing when they first occurred?
• Ask if anything aggravates the symptom or relieves it.
• Does he have any associated symptoms, such as dizziness or weakness?
• Does he drink beverages containing caffeine, such as cola or coffee?

Analyzing the chief complaint. Defined as a patient's conscious awareness of his own heartbeat, palpitations may be reported as an uncomfortable, strange feeling in the chest. Patients may say their heart is beating fast or irregularly, pounding, or skipping beats. The palpitations may be regular or irregular, fast or slow, paroxysmal or sustained. Usually occurring at the cardiac apex, palpitations may also be felt substernally or in the neck.

Frequently insignificant, transient palpitations can result from smoking, exercise, stress, or excessive caffeine intake. Nonpathologic palpitations may also occur with a newly implanted prosthetic valve because its clicking sound heightens the patient's awareness of his heartbeat.

Paroxysmal or sustained palpitations—accompanied by dizziness; weakness; fatigue; an irregular, rapid, or slow pulse; and decreased blood pressure—may signal cardiac arrhythmias.

Mitral valve prolapse may cause paroxysmal palpitations accompanied by sharp, stabbing, or aching precordial pain. Early features of mitral valve disease include sustained palpitations with dyspnea and fatigue on exertion.

Fatigue. If your patient complains of fatigue, explore his problem by asking appropriate questions from this list.
• What activity causes him to feel fatigued? How long can he perform this activity before he tires?
• Does rest relieve the fatigue?
• Does he feel more tired now than he did 2 months ago?

Analyzing the chief complaint. A feeling of excessive tiredness, lack of energy, or exhaustion accompanied by a strong desire to rest or sleep, fatigue is a normal response to physical overexertion, prolonged

Causes of chest pain

When a patient experiences chest pain, you may first suspect a cardiac cause. Use this chart to differentiate cardiac-related chest pain from other types of chest pain.

CAUSE AND CHARACTERISTICS	LOCATION	INFLUENCING FACTORS
Heart		
Angina pectoris Aching, squeezing, pressure, heaviness, burning; usually subsides within 10 minutes; unstable angina appears even at rest	Substernal area; may radiate to jaw, neck, arms, and back	*Aggravating:* Eating, exertion, smoking, cold, stress, anger, hunger, lying down *Alleviating:* Rest, nitroglycerin
Acute myocardial infarction Pressure, burning, aching, tightness; diaphoresis, weakness, anxiety, nausea; sudden onset; lasts ½ hour to 2 hours	Across chest; may radiate to jaw, neck, arms, and back	*Aggravating:* Exertion, anxiety *Alleviating:* Analgesics, particularly morphine sulfate
Pericarditis Sharp; may be accompanied by pleural friction rub; sudden onset; continuous pain	Substernal area; radiating to neck and left arm	*Aggravating:* Deep breathing, supine position *Alleviating:* Sitting up, leaning forward, anti-inflammatory agents
Dissecting aortic aneurysm Excruciating, tearing; possible blood pressure difference between right and left arms; sudden onset	Retrosternal area, upper abdomen, or epigastrium; radiating to back, neck, and shoulders	*Aggravating:* None *Alleviating:* Analgesics, but emergency surgery is usually indicated
Lung		
Pulmonary embolus Sudden, knifelike; cyanosis, dyspnea, or cough with hemoptysis	Over lung area	*Aggravating:* Inspiration *Alleviating:* Analgesics
Pneumothorax Unilateral, sudden, severe, and increases with movement; dyspnea, increased pulse rate, decreased or absent breath sounds, deviated trachea	Lateral thorax	*Aggravating:* Normal respiration *Alleviating:* Analgesics, chest tube
Abdomen		
Esophageal spasm Dull, pressurelike, squeezing	Substernal area, epigastrium	*Aggravating:* Food, cold liquids, exercise *Alleviating:* Nitroglycerin, calcium channel blockers

Causes of chest pain *(continued)*

CAUSE AND CHARACTERISTICS	LOCATION	INFLUENCING FACTORS
Hiatal hernia Sharp, severe	Lower chest, upper abdomen	*Aggravating:* Heavy meal, bending, lying down *Alleviating:* Antacids, walking, semi-Fowler's position
Peptic ulcer Burning after eating; hematemesis or tarry stools; sudden onset, usually subsides in 15 to 20 minutes	Epigastrium	*Aggravating:* Lack of food or highly acidic foods *Alleviating:* Food, antacids
Cholecystitis Gripping, sharp; possible nausea and vomiting	Right epigastrium or abdomen; radiating to shoulders	*Aggravating:* Fatty foods, lying down *Alleviating:* Rest, analgesics, surgery
Other		
Chest wall syndrome Sharp; tender to the touch; gradual or sudden onset; continuous or intermittent	Anywhere in chest	*Aggravating:* Movement, palpation *Alleviating:* Time, analgesics, heat
Acute anxiety Dull, stabbing; hyperventilation or dyspnea; sudden onset; transient or may last for several days	Anywhere in chest	*Aggravating:* Increased respiratory rate, stress or anxiety *Alleviating:* Slowing of respiratory rate, stress relief

emotional stress, and sleep deprivation. Persistent fatigue can also be a nonspecific symptom of a physiologic disorder such as CHF, although few patients recognize fatigue as a cardiac symptom. Usually, when a patient feels fatigued during an activity, he stops to rest, often preventing the more obvious cardiac symptoms.

All types of valvular heart disease commonly produce progressive fatigue. In MI, fatigue can be severe but will probably be overshadowed by chest pain. In a patient receiving cardiac glycoside therapy, fatigue may indicate toxicity.

Edema. If your patient complains of edema, explore his problem by asking appropriate questions from this list.
• Ask him to point to where the swelling occurs.
• Is there a particular time of day when the swelling occurs or worsens? Does anything relieve it?
• Is the swelling associated with any other symptoms?
• How long has he had this problem?

Analyzing the chief complaint. When associated with cardiac problems, edema may be chronic and progressive. It usually results from increased capillary hydrostatic pressure, which displaces fluid from the capillaries into the tissues. This causes a visibly excessive accumulation of interstitial fluid. Cardiac-related edema may accompany hypertension, left ventricular failure, and increased venous pressure secondary to right heart failure.

In pericardial effusion, generalized pitting edema may be most prominent in the arms and legs. It may be accompanied by chest pain, dyspnea, nonproductive cough, dysphagia, and fever.

In CHF, severe, generalized pitting edema may follow leg edema late in the disorder. The edema may improve with exercise or elevation of the limbs and may be accompanied by tachypnea, palpitations, hypotension, and weight gain despite anorexia.

Physical assessment

Inspection and, especially, auscultation form the cornerstone of the heart examination. Usually, palpation and percussion aren't warranted in a rapid assessment. If they are, perform them after you auscultate. During the examination, keep in mind the basic anatomy of the heart, along with the normal assessment findings. (See *Heart: Normal findings*.)

Inspection. To inspect the precordium, first place the patient supine with his head flat or elevated for his respiratory comfort. Standing to his right (unless you're left-handed), remove the clothing covering his chest wall and quickly identify the following anatomic sites, named for their underlying structures: the sternoclavicular, pulmonary, aortic, right ventricular, epigastric, and left ventricular areas. Make a visual sweep

of the chest wall, watching for movement, pulsations, and exaggerated lifts or heaves (strong outward thrusts over the chest during systole).

If you're examining an obese patient or one with large breasts, have the patient sit upright. This will bring the heart closer to the anterior chest wall and make any pulsations more visible. If time allows, you can use tangential lighting to cast shadows across the chest. This makes it easier to see any abnormalities.

During your inspection, consider any visible pulsation to the right of the sternum abnormal; this may indicate an aortic aneurysm. A pulsation in the sternoclavicular or epigastric areas also may indicate an aortic aneurysm. A sustained, forceful apical impulse suggests left ventricular hypertrophy, which is associated with high blood pressure and may cause cardiomyopathy and mitral regurgitation. A laterally displaced apical impulse may be a sign of left ventricular hypertrophy or aortic stenosis.

Auscultation. You'll find auscultation the most important assessment tool in evaluating the heart. Using a stethoscope with a 10″ to 12″ (25- to 30-cm) tube, auscultate over the precordium to detect heart sounds (see *Identifying auscultatory sites*, page 116).

Normal heart sounds. Place the diaphragm of the stethoscope at the apex of the heart to identify the heart's rate, rhythm, and normal sounds — the S_1 and the S_2 sounds. If heart sounds are faint or undetectable — possibly from a thick chest wall — try moving the patient from a supine position to a semi-Fowler's position. If heart sounds are still

CHECKLIST

Heart: Normal findings

Inspection
Normal findings include:
☐ no visible pulsations, except at the point of maximal impulse (PMI).
☐ no lifts (heaves) or retractions in the four valve areas of the chest wall.

Auscultation
Normal findings include:
☐ an S_1 sound—the "lub" sound heard best with the diaphragm of the stethoscope over the mitral area with the patient in a left lateral position. It sounds longer, lower, and louder there than S_2 sounds. S_1 splitting may be audible in the tricuspid area.
☐ an S_2 sound—the "dub" sound heard best through the diaphragm of the stethoscope in the aortic area with the patient sitting and leaning over. It sounds shorter, sharper, higher, and louder there than S_1. Normal S_2 splitting may be audible on inspiration in the pulmonary area.
☐ an S_3 sound; in children and slen-

der, young adults with no cardiovascular disease, S_3 is normal. S_3 may be heard best with the bell of the stethoscope over the mitral area with the patient supine and exhaling. It sounds short, dull, soft, and low.
☐ murmurs; may be functional in children and young adults. Innocent murmurs are soft, short, and vary with respirations and patient position. They occur in early systole and are heard best in pulmonary or mitral areas with the patient supine.

Palpation
Normal findings include:
☐ no detectable vibrations or thrills
☐ no lifts
☐ no pulsations, except at the PMI and epigastric area. At PMI, a localized ($<$ ½" [1.25-cm] diameter area) tapping pulse may be felt at the start of systole. In the epigastric area, pulsation from the abdominal aorta may be palpable.

faint, the patient may have cardiac tamponade. A left lateral decubitus position may make it easier for you to hear low-pitched sounds related to atrioventricular valve problems.

Ventricular gallop. Using the bell of the stethoscope, you may hear S_3 sounds, or ventricular gallops, early in diastole. These sounds develop from vibrations that occur during rapid, early ventricular filling into a dilated ventricle. Although ventricular gallops are normal in children and some young, slender adults with no cardiovascular disease, they're pathologic in most adults.

Ventricular gallops normally strengthen with movements that increase venous return and disappear when the rapid-filling disorder resolves. A sign of CHF, ventricular gallops may stem from mitral regurgitation, acute left ventricular failure, or hypertension. They also may occur in conditions causing volume overload and ventricular dilation, such as mitral, aortic, or tricuspid insufficiency. With right-sided S_3, suspect right ventricular failure, pulmonary embolism, or pulmonary hypertension.

Atrial gallop. The S_4, or atrial gallop, may result from atrial kick—the vibrations occurring in late diastole after blood flows from the atrium into the ventricle with decreased compliance. This sound, heard with the bell of the stethoscope, fre-

Identifying auscultatory sites

When auscultating the precordium, listen for each heart sound, moving the stethoscope slowly over the five main anatomic areas shown below.

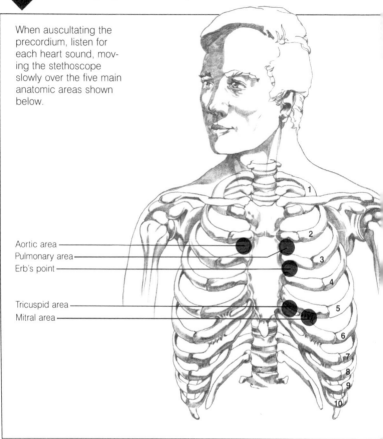

Aortic area
Pulmonary area
Erb's point
Tricuspid area
Mitral area

quently indicates systemic hypertension, CAD, cardiomyopathy, or severe aortic stenosis. Right-sided S_4 may be heard best along the lower left sternal border. Although S_4 usually indicates cardiac disease, you may hear it in a patient with a normal heart. A summation gallop may develop when a rapid heart rate fuses S_3 and S_4. Arising in mid-diastole, this sound may best be heard at the cardiac apex.

Pericardial friction rub. If you suspect pericarditis, listen with your stethoscope diaphragm for a pericardial friction rub (a scratchy sound produced when the parietal and visceral surfaces of the pericardium rub against each other). You may hear the sound anywhere along the left anterior chest, but you'll probably hear it best at the tricuspid valve area. Have the patient lean forward and exhale forcefully so you can listen after exhalation, without the sound of expiration interfering. You should be able to hear the sound during systole and diastole, but remember that pericardial friction rubs can be intermittent.

Further assessment. As with the lungs, you may need to assess other body areas — either to gather additional information or to confirm your findings. For instance, you may want to assess the lungs because cardiac-related symptoms often result from a respiratory disorder.

As appropriate, you may also assess the following:
• the fingers for clubbing — a sign of chronic heart disease and consequently prolonged hypoxemia
• the peripheral pulses; the rate and rhythm may reveal a problem in cardiac function and peripheral perfusion
• the neck for jugular vein distention, carotid pulse, and bruits
• the face, arms, and legs for signs of edema, which may indicate increased hydrostatic pressure
• the nail beds for cyanosis
• the mucous membranes of the mouth and the lips for cyanosis.

After obtaining a history and performing the physical assessment, you'll begin to form a diagnostic impression (see *Heart: Interpreting your findings*, pages 118 to 120).

Pediatric considerations

When you rapidly assess the heart of an infant or a child, modify your assessment technique to accommodate developmental differences. Assess the child's developmental stage. Since cardiovascular dysfunction can retard development, you'll need to evaluate his height, weight, growth pattern, and motor and cognitive abilities. During the examination, look for ways to allay the

patient's anxiety, as well as that of his parents.

Vital signs. When checking a pediatric patient's pulse rate, keep in mind that the normal value varies according to age. For example, a neonate's pulse rate may range between 70 and 130. As the child gets older, his pulse rate gradually decreases to adult levels.

A neonate's blood pressure normally will be much lower than that of an adult and will increase with age. When taking an infant's or child's blood pressure, make sure you use the appropriate cuff size. And remember, since blood pressure may be inaudible in children under age 2, consider using an electronic stethoscope to get a more accurate measurement.

Inspection. Pallor can indicate a serious cardiac disorder in an infant or anemia in an older child. And cyanosis may be an early sign of a cardiac condition. Cyanosis of the extremities is a common and often normal finding in neonates but still requires evaluation.

When checking for finger clubbing, remember that it doesn't ordinarily occur before age 2. Also remember that dependent edema, a late sign of CHF, appears in the legs only if the child can walk; in infants, it appears in the eyelids. If the child is bedridden, make sure you check both his sacrum and buttocks for edema.

Auscultation. In many normal, healthy children, auscultation reveals a split S_2. Splitting occurs during inspiration, when right ventricular ejection takes slightly longer than left ventricular ejection. This results in a slight delay in the

(Text continues on page 120.)

DIAGNOSTIC IMPRESSION

Heart: Interpreting your findings

After you assess the patient, a group of findings may lead you to suspect a particular disorder. The chart below shows you some common groups of findings for the chief complaints of the heart, along with the appropriate nursing diagnostic categories and probable causes.

CHIEF COMPLAINT AND FINDINGS	NURSING DIAGNOSTIC CATEGORIES	PROBABLE CAUSE
Chest pain		
• Sudden, constricting or crushing chest pain unrelieved by nitroglycerin or rest; typically affects the central and substernal area but may radiate to the left arm, jaw, neck, or shoulder blades • Anxiety, tenseness, sense of impending doom • Clammy skin • Crackles • Diaphoresis • Distant sounding gallop rhythm • Dyspnea • Nausea • Normal or decreased blood pressure • Pallor or cyanosis • Pericardial friction rub • Restlessness • Tachycardia or bradycardia and weak pulse • Weakness	• Activity intolerance • Altered sexuality patterns • Anxiety • Decreased cardiac output • Fear (of pain, death) • Pain • Potential body image disturbance • Sleep pattern disturbance	Myocardial infarction
• Gradual onset; feeling of tightness, aching, burning, squeezing, pressure; radiates to neck, jaw; provoked by ambulation, relieved by nitroglycerin • Anxiety • Sensation of indigestion in retrosternal region	• Activity intolerance • Anxiety • Decreased cardiac output • Fear • Knowledge deficit • Pain • Potential self-care deficit	Angina
Dyspnea		
• Dyspnea arises suddenly and progressively worsens • Anxiety • Cool, clammy skin • Decreased mental acuity • Decreased peripheral pulses • Restlessness • Severe hypotension • Tachycardia • Tachypnea	• Altered cardiopulmonary tissue perfusion • Altered cerebral tissue perfusion • Altered peripheral tissue perfusion • Anxiety • Fear • Impaired gas exchange	Shock

DIAGNOSTIC IMPRESSION

Heart: Interpreting your findings *(continued)*

CHIEF COMPLAINT AND FINDINGS	NURSING DIAGNOSTIC CATEGORIES	PROBABLE CAUSE
Dyspnea		
• Dyspnea occurs on exertion and at rest • Orthopnea • Paroxysmal nocturnal dyspnea • Fatigue that increases as exercise tolerance decreases • Flushed cheeks • Hemoptysis • Localized; delayed, rumbling, low-pitched murmur at or near apex • Mid-diastolic or presystolic thrill (or both) at apex • Pain in extremities • Precordial bulge and diffuse pulsation in young patient • Weak pulse • Tapping sensation over normal area of apical impulse	• Activity intolerance • Fatigue • Ineffective breathing pattern • Pain • Sleep pattern disturbance	Mitral stenosis
Paroxysmal palpitations		
• Dizziness • Dyspnea • Mid-systolic click, followed by a late, high-pitched apical systolic murmur • Paroxysmal tachycardia • Severe fatigue • Sharp, stabbing or aching precordial pain	• Anxiety • Fatigue • Pain	Mitral prolapse
Nonparoxysmal palpitations		
• Anxiety • Diaphoresis • Facial flushing • Hyperventilation leading to dizziness, weakness, and syncope • Trembling	• Anxiety • Fear • Potential for injury • Potential impaired gas exchange	Acute anxiety attack
Fatigue		
• Bounding pulse • Dyspnea • Pallor • Systolic bruit over carotid artery • Tachycardia	• Altered cardiopulmonary tissue perfusion • Altered peripheral tissue perfusion • Fatigue • Impaired gas exchange	Anemia

(continued)

DIAGNOSTIC IMPRESSION

Heart: Interpreting your findings *(continued)*

CHIEF COMPLAINT AND FINDINGS	NURSING DIAGNOSTIC CATEGORIES	PROBABLE CAUSE
Fatigue		
• Daytime oliguria • Exertional and paroxysmal nocturnal dyspnea • Heaving apical impulse • Lethargy • Pallor or cyanosis • S_3 and S_4 heart sounds • Tachycardia • Weakness • Weight gain • Wheezing on inspiration and expiration	• Activity intolerance • Decreased cardiac output • Fatigue • Ineffective breathing pattern • Sleep pattern disturbance	Left ventricular failure
Edema		
• Dependent edema beginning in ankles and progressing to legs and genitalia • Abdominal fluid wave and shifting dullness • Anorexia • Dyspnea • Fatigue • Jugular vein distention • Lower left sternal heave, independent of apical impulse • Nausea, vomiting • Palpation reveals enlarged, tender, pulsating liver • Right upper abdominal pain upon exertion • Right ventricular S_3 sound • Tachycardia • Tricuspid regurgitation murmur • Weight gain	• Activity intolerance • Fatigue • Fluid volume excess • Ineffective breathing pattern • Pain	Right ventricular failure

pulmonary valve closing.

The inspiratory delay is long enough to allow you to discriminate two separate components of S_2, which sound like "di-dub" and reflect the aortic and pulmonary valve closings. Splitting is less likely to occur during expiration because the semilunar valves close more synchronously, but it can occur with arrhythmias, septal defects, and pulmonary disease.

Palpation. In a child under age 4, expect to find the point of maximal impulse (PMI) at the third or fourth intercostal space. In older children, you'll find the PMI at the fifth intercostal space. A displaced PMI in a child suggests coarctation of the aorta.

Geriatric considerations

You'll use the same assessment techniques for elderly patients as you would for any adult, but the findings may vary because of normal age-related changes. An elderly patient may be less likely to notice changes in his baseline status. Instead, he may simply become less active to compensate for any problems, making accurate heart assessment more difficult.

An elderly patient also may have an increased pain threshold, which affects his ability to interpret symptoms. For example, if a patient sustains an MI, he may tell you he feels short of breath or that he doesn't feel well.

An elderly patient who has CHF may have ankle edema, be confused, and lose his appetite, but have no other specific symptoms. Keep in mind, too, that many elderly people take medications that can produce various cardiovascular effects. For example, certain antiarthritic drugs may cause fluid retention and edema.

Vital signs. As the body ages, the heart rate slows and the blood pressure increases to a level between 140/70 and 160/90 mm Hg. Although the systolic and diastolic blood pressures both increase, the systolic pressure rise is greater because of the increased rigidity of the vascular tree.

Inspection. During your inspection of the sternoclavicular area, you may detect obvious pulsations that are caused by calcification and dilation of the aorta. If so, you'll also note that the superficial vessels of the forehead, neck, and extremities will feel prominent and ropelike on palpation.

Auscultation. Because the chest is more likely to be deformed in an elderly patient, you may find auscultation difficult. These deformities may be secondary to kyphosis, scoliosis, kyphoscoliosis, and old compression fractures that make the bony chest shorter. The chest may also be barrel-shaped.

Kyphosis and scoliosis also distort the chest walls and may displace the heart slightly. Thus, your patient's PMI and heart sounds may be displaced. These deformities increase the distance that heart sounds must cross, making their interpretation more difficult. To increase the intensity of heart sounds, have an elderly patient sit up or lean forward during auscultation, if possible.

Suggested readings

Bates, B. *A Guide to Physical Examination and History Taking.* Philadelphia: J.B. Lippincott Co., 1987.

Becker, K.L., and Stevens, S.A. "Get in Touch and in Tune with Cardiac Assessment," Part 1. *Nursing88* 18(3):51-55, March 1988.

Cardiopulmonary Emergencies. Springhouse, Pa.: Springhouse Corp., 1991.

Donner, C., and Cooper, K. "The Critical Difference: Pulmonary Edema," *American Journal of Nursing* 88(1):59, January 1988.

Ellstrom, K. "What's Causing Your Patient's Respiratory Distress?" *Nursing90* 20(11):57-61, November 1990.

Engel, J. *Pocket Nurse Guide to Pediatric Assessment.* St. Louis: C.V. Mosby Co., 1989.

Handerhan, B. "Action Stat! Chest Pain," *Nursing89* 19(6):33, June 1989.

Illustrated Manual of Nursing Practice.

Springhouse, Pa.: Springhouse Corp., 1991.

Lanros, N.E. *Assessment and Intervention in Emergency Nursing,* 3rd ed. East Norwalk, Conn.: Appleton & Lange, 1988.

Malasanos, L., et al. *Health Assessment,* 4th ed. St. Louis: C.V. Mosby Co., 1989.

Metzgar, E.D., and Stinger, K.A. *Health Assessment: A Study and Learning Tool.* Springhouse Notes Series. Springhouse, Pa.: Springhouse Corporation, 1988.

Morton, P.G. *Health Assessment in Nursing.* Springhouse, Pa.: Springhouse Corporation, 1989.

Raisch, P., and Klaus, B.J. *Every Nurse's Guide to Physical Assessment: A Primary Focus.* New York: John Wiley & Sons, 1987.

Stevens, S.A., and Becker, K.L. "How to Perform Picture-Perfect Respiratory Assessment," *Nursing88* 18(1):57-63, January 1988.

Swartz, M.H. *Textbook of Physical Diagnosis: History and Examination.* Philadelphia: W.B. Saunders Co., 1989.

Weber, J., ed. *Nurse's Handbook of Health Assessment.* Philadelphia: J.B. Lippincott Co., 1988.

6

ASSESSMENT
OF THE
ABDOMEN

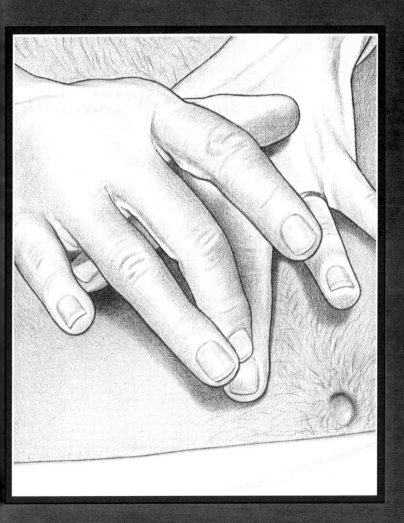

Abdominal complaints can be especially difficult to assess. That's because the abdomen houses so many organs and structures—including the GI system (stomach, intestines, liver, pancreas, gallbladder), urinary system (kidneys, ureters, bladder), and reproductive system (ovaries and uterus in women, prostate in men).

But accurate rapid assessment is critical. For abdominal complaints not only are common, they also frequently point to serious—and sometimes life-threatening—problems, many of which develop quickly.

This chapter spells out what you need to know to perform a rapid abdominal assessment of an adult. It describes how to pinpoint the nature of the patient's chief complaint and evaluate its seriousness, using critical health history questions. Then the chapter covers the streamlined techniques you'll use to inspect, auscultate, percuss, and palpate the abdomen. Finally, you'll find a discussion of the special considerations that affect abdominal assessment of pediatric and elderly patients.

Remember that depending on your findings, you may have to interrupt your abdominal assessment to examine another part of the body. Or you may need to stop your assessment to intervene in an emergency.

Abdomen

Accurate, rapid abdominal assessment depends on a well-focused health history and physical examination. But first you must make some general observations and measure your patient's vital signs. (See *Reviewing abdominal structures.*)

General observations

Quickly survey the entire abdomen for visible deformities and observe the patient for obvious signs of nutritional problems, such as cachexia or extreme obesity. If time and the patient's condition permit, weigh him.

Note the patient's level of consciousness (LOC). Also note his facial expression, body movements, posture, and skin condition for clues to his overall health status.

Level of consciousness. Assess the patient's LOC. In certain critical conditions, such as hemorrhage or perforation, decreasing LOC indicates the need for immediate intervention.

Face and body. Observe the patient's facial expression, body movements, and posture for signs of distress. Watch for signs of pain such as grimacing, writhing, clutching the abdomen, or assuming a rigid or hunched-over position. Also watch for frequent position changes, which may indicate attempts to relieve pain or discomfort.

Skin condition. Assess the patient's skin, noting color, integrity, and turgor. Pallor, diaphoresis, and cool, clammy skin may indicate internal hemorrhage. If you note these findings, quickly assess his vital signs, notify the doctor, and prepare to take immediate action. Dry skin and mucous membranes with poor skin turgor may indicate dehydration, requiring fluid and electrolyte replacement therapy. Jaundice, a yellowish discoloration of the skin or mucous membranes, may point to hepatic damage or biliary obstruction.

Vital signs

As soon as possible, obtain vital

Reviewing abdominal structures

This illustration shows the normal position of the abdominal structures.

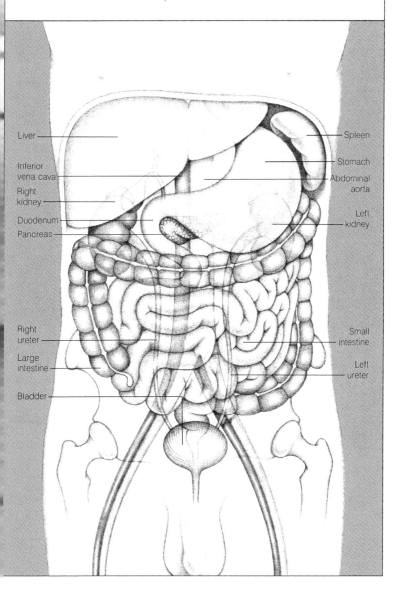

Liver

Inferior
vena cava

Right
kidney

Duodenum

Pancreas

Right
ureter

Large
intestine

Bladder

Spleen

Stomach

Abdominal
aorta

Left
kidney

Small
intestine

Left
ureter

signs to establish a baseline. Then periodically monitor vital signs for changes that may signal hemodynamic alterations or an infectious process — both of which commonly affect the abdomen.

Temperature. Accurate temperature readings can help detect an early onset of fever, an important sign of infection or inflammation.

Pulse. Tachycardia may occur with shock, pain, fever, sepsis, fluid overload, or anxiety. A weak, rapid, and irregular pulse may point to hemodynamic instability, such as that caused by excessive blood loss. Diminished or absent distal pulses may signal vessel occlusion from embolization associated with prolonged bleeding.

Respirations. Altered respiratory rate and depth can result from hypoxia, pain, electrolyte imbalance, or anxiety. As with blood pressure and pulse, respiratory rate initially increases with shock. Increased respiratory rate with shallow respirations may signal fever and sepsis. Absent or shallow abdominal movement on respiration may point to peritoneal irritation.

Blood pressure. If time permits, measure blood pressure in both arms for comparison. Also, measure blood pressure with the patient lying down and sitting up, if possible.

Decreased blood pressure may signal compromised hemodynamic status — perhaps from shock caused by GI hemorrhage. Sustained, severe hypotension (systolic pressure below 70 mm Hg) results in diminished renal blood flow, which may lead to acute renal failure. Moderately increased systolic or diastolic pressure may occur with anxiety or abdominal pain. Hypertension can result from vascular damage caused by renal disease or renal artery stenosis. A blood pressure drop of greater than 30 mm Hg when the patient sits up may indicate fluid volume depletion.

History
After completing your general observations and vital signs check, obtain a quick history of the patient's chief complaint. Significant complaints include abdominal pain, nausea and vomiting, diarrhea, constipation, changes in voiding patterns, rectal bleeding, and abnormal vaginal bleeding.

Abdominal pain. If the patient complains of abdominal pain, explore his problem by asking appropriate questions from this list.
• When did the patient first notice the pain? What was he doing when it started? Ask if it started slowly or suddenly.
• Have the patient describe the pain. Is it sharp, dull, burning, aching, squeezing, or cramping?
• Where exactly is the pain? Does it spread to other areas? Have the patient show you, if possible. Also ask when and how the pain occurs. Is it constant or intermittent? More pronounced at certain times of the day or night? Does the pain awaken him? How long does it last?
• Has the pain gotten worse or better, or stayed the same? Does anything relieve or aggravate it — for example, activity, eating, urinating, defecating, or changing position?
• Ask about any accompanying signs or symptoms, such as loss of appetite, indigestion, nausea, vomiting, diarrhea, constipation, change in stool color, rectal bleeding, fever, weight loss, or yellowish skin color.

Abdominal pain: Types and locations

AFFECTED ORGAN	VISCERAL PAIN	SOMATIC PAIN	REFERRED PAIN
Stomach	Middle epigastrium	Middle epigastrium and left upper quadrant	Shoulders
Small intestine	Periumbilical area	Over affected site	Midback (rare)
Appendix	Periumbilical area	Right lower quadrant	Right lower quadrant
Proximal colon	Periumbilical area and right flank for ascending colon	Over affected site	Right lower quadrant and back (rare)
Distal colon	Hypogastrium and left flank for descending colon	Over affected site	Left lower quadrant and back (rare)
Gallbladder	Middle epigastrium	Right upper quadrant	Right subscapular area
Ureters	Costovertebral angle	Over affected site	Groin; scrotum in men, labia in women (rare)
Pancreas	Middle epigastrium and left upper quadrant	Middle epigastrium and left upper quadrant	Back and left shoulder
Ovaries, fallopian tubes, and uterus	Hypogastrium and groin	Over affected site	Inner thighs

Also ask about urinary frequency, urgency, burning, menstrual irregularities, dyspareunia, or vaginal or penile discharge.

• Has the patient taken any over-the-counter or prescription drugs to relieve the abdominal pain? If so, what did he take and how often did he take it?

Analyzing the chief complaint. A highly subjective symptom, abdominal pain can be described in widely varying ways. Patients may report "indigestion," "heartburn," "stomachache," or other such nonspecific complaints that require careful investigation. A patient experiencing diffuse pain may be unable to locate its exact source. In contrast, another patient may be able to locate his pain and describe any radiation to other body areas. (See *Abdominal pain: Types and locations.*)

Abdominal pain may arise from the abdominopelvic viscera, the parietal peritoneum, or the capsules of the liver, kidney, or spleen. Visceral pain develops slowly into a poorly localized dull ache. In contrast, somatic pain, caused by inflammation usually originating in the peritoneum, produces a sharp, more intense, and well-localized discomfort

Causes of abdominal pain

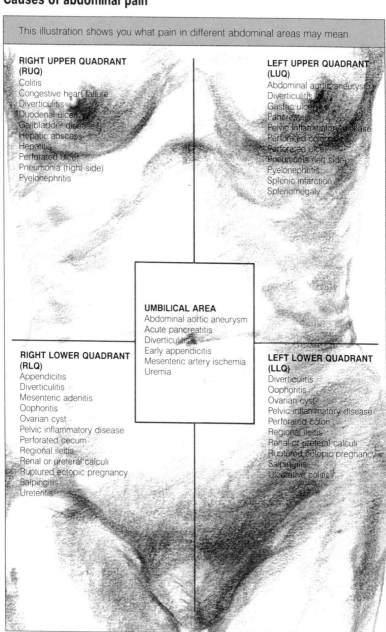

This illustration shows you what pain in different abdominal areas may mean.

RIGHT UPPER QUADRANT (RUQ)
Colitis
Congestive heart failure
Diverticulitis
Duodenal ulcer
Gallbladder disease
Hepatic abscess
Hepatitis
Perforated ulcer
Pneumonia (right side)
Pyelonephritis

LEFT UPPER QUADRANT (LUQ)
Abdominal aortic aneurysm
Diverticulitis
Gastric ulcer
Pancreatitis
Pelvic inflammatory disease
Perforated colon
Perforated ulcer
Pneumonia (left side)
Pyelonephritis
Splenic infarction
Splenomegaly

UMBILICAL AREA
Abdominal aortic aneurysm
Acute pancreatitis
Diverticulitis
Early appendicitis
Mesenteric artery ischemia
Uremia

RIGHT LOWER QUADRANT (RLQ)
Appendicitis
Diverticulitis
Mesenteric adenitis
Oophoritis
Ovarian cyst
Pelvic inflammatory disease
Perforated cecum
Regional ileitis
Renal or ureteral calculi
Ruptured ectopic pregnancy
Salpingitis
Ureteritis

LEFT LOWER QUADRANT (LLQ)
Diverticulitis
Oophoritis
Ovarian cyst
Pelvic inflammatory disease
Perforated colon
Regional ileitis
Renal or ureteral calculi
Ruptured ectopic pregnancy
Salpingitis
Ulcerative colitis

that rapidly follows an injury. Movement or coughing aggravates this pain.

Pain may be referred from the abdomen to distant sites, or to the abdomen from another site with the same or similar nerve supply. This sharp, well-localized pain is felt in skin or deeper tissues and may coexist with skin hyperesthesia and muscular hyperalgesia.

Usually, abdominal pain results from GI disorders, such as pancreatitis, gastritis, gastroenteritis, cholecystitis, intestinal obstruction, appendicitis, irritable bowel syndrome, and ulcer disease. (See *Causes of abdominal pain.*) But abdominal pain can also result from:
• reproductive disorders, such as ectopic pregnancy, endometriosis, pelvic inflammatory disease, and ovarian cysts
• genitourinary disorders, such as cystitis, pyelonephritis, prostatitis, and renal calculi
• musculoskeletal problems, such as abdominal muscular or bone disorders
• cardiovascular disorders, such as abdominal aortic aneurysm, myocardial infarction, congestive heart failure, angina, and mesenteric artery ischemia
• drugs, such as salicylates and non-steroidal anti-inflammatory drugs
• toxins, such as insect stings and amebiasis.

The duration of abdominal pain provides an important clue to its cause. Constant, steady pain suggests organ perforation, ischemia, inflammation, or blood accumulation in the peritoneal cavity. Conversely, intermittent, cramping pain points to hollow organ (such as bowel) obstruction.

Pain in the area from the lower ribs to the ileum can indicate upper urinary tract disease or trauma.

Such pain is commonly aggravated by costovertebral angle (CVA) percussion and, in patients with renal or urinary tract obstruction, by increased fluid intake or ingestion of alcohol, caffeine, or diuretic drugs.

In a pregnant patient, acute abdominal pain may signal a complication of pregnancy. If a pregnant patient complains of abdominal pain, you should notify the doctor immediately.

Nausea and vomiting. If the patient complains of nausea and vomiting, explore his problem by asking appropriate questions from this list.
• When did the patient first experience these symptoms? Did the nausea precede the vomiting? If so, how long after he felt nauseated did he vomit? Was the vomiting projectile?
• Does anything seem to help relieve the nausea and vomiting? Does anything make it worse?
• When was the last time he felt nauseated or vomited? How often does it occur?
• Have the patient describe the color, odor, and appearance of the vomitus. Does it contain any undigested food or blood? If so, how much?
• Ask the patient about his appetite. Does he notice any increase or decrease? Is the nausea or vomiting associated with eating or drinking? If so, does any specific food or drink seem to cause it?
• Does a particular activity or change in position affect the nausea and vomiting?
• Ask about related symptoms, such as abdominal pain, anorexia, changes in bowel habits or stool appearance, excessive belching, flatus or a sense of bloating, or indigestion. Has he noticed a recent weight loss? If so, how much?

• Ask a premenopausal patient when she had her last menstrual period. Is there a possibility that she's pregnant?

Analyzing the chief complaint. A sensation of profound revulsion to food or of impending vomiting, nausea commonly accompanies autonomic nervous system changes, such as hypersalivation, diaphoresis, tachycardia, pallor, and tachypnea. Nausea is closely linked to vomiting, the forceful expulsion of gastric contents through the mouth. Characteristically preceded by nausea, vomiting results from a coordinated sequence of abdominal muscle contractions and reverse esophageal peristalsis.

Nausea and vomiting are common complaints associated with food poisoning and with GI disorders, such as acute cholecystitis, appendicitis, intestinal obstruction, peritonitis, ulcers, and gastroenteritis. These two symptoms can also occur with:
• fluid and electrolyte disorders, such as hyponatremia, hypernatremia, hypokalemia, and hypercalcemia
• intestinal infections
• metabolic disorders such as metabolic acidosis
• endocrine disorders, such as adrenal insufficiency and thyrotoxicosis
• labyrinthine disorders, such as Ménière's disease and labyrinthitis
• cardiovascular disorders, such as congestive heart failure, mesenteric artery thrombosis, mesenteric venous thrombosis, and myocardial infarction
• renal disorders, such as cystitis, pyelonephritis, and renal calculi
• reproductive conditions, such as hyperemesis gravidarum and pregnancy-induced hypertension
• drugs, such as antineoplastic agents, opiates, and antibiotics
• radiation therapy and surgery, especially abdominal surgery
• severe pain, stress, anxiety, alcohol intoxication, overeating, and ingestion of distasteful foods or liquids.

Nausea and vomiting commonly occur during the first trimester of pregnancy. However, vomiting in later stages of pregnancy can signal complications.

Vomiting also may point to central nervous system problems. For example, projectile vomiting not preceded by nausea is a cardinal sign of increased intracranial pressure.

In GI disorders, vomiting may indicate severe peritoneal irritation resulting from a perforated abdominal organ, ingestion of toxins, or obstruction of the intestine, ureter, or bile duct. Vomiting associated with perforation usually isn't severe. In obstruction, vomiting commonly occurs with severe pain; with an intestinal obstruction, it's often bilious initially, followed by fluid with a fecal odor. Biliary colic also produces bilious vomitus.

Other characteristics of the vomitus may provide important clues to the cause of vomiting. For instance, bloody vomitus may indicate upper GI bleeding, as from gastritis, peptic ulcer, or esophageal or gastric varices. Coffee-ground vomitus contains digested blood such as from a slowly bleeding gastric or duodenal lesion. Vomitus containing undigested food may indicate a gastric outlet obstruction. (See *Vomitus: Characteristics and causes.*)

Remember, vomiting calls for immediate intervention if it's prolonged, associated with hematemesis, or projectile and unaccompanied by nausea. Also be prepared to intervene if the patient is at risk for aspiration.

iarrhea. If the patient complains of ...arrhea, explore his problem by ...king appropriate questions from ...is list.

Ask about the onset of diarrhea. ...as it sudden or gradual? When did ...begin, and what was the patient ...ping before it started?

How often does diarrhea occur? ...ow often today? Does it seem ...orse at a particular time of day? ...pes anything seem to relieve it? ...ggravate it?

Have the patient describe the diar-...ea (amount, consistency, color, ...d odor). Is the stool bloody, dark ...ack, bulky, foul-smelling, or ...easy?

What foods did he eat before the ...set of diarrhea? Has he traveled ...cently? Ask about related symp-...ms, such as abdominal pain, ...amping, nausea, or vomiting.

How often does he normally have ...bowel movement? Do periods of ...nstipation alternate with periods of ...diarrhea?

Does the patient take any laxatives ...other medications? If so, what ...nd and how often?

nalyzing the chief complaint. Com-...only signaling an intestinal disor-...r, diarrhea varies in severity and ...ay be acute or chronic. Periods of ...arrhea alternating with periods of ...nstipation may indicate irritable ...wel syndrome, diverticulitis, colo-...ctal cancer, or Crohn's disease. ...ute diarrhea accompanied by ...amping and vomiting may point to ...od poisoning. Fever, tenesmus, ...d cramping associated with acute ...arrhea usually indicate a viral in-...ction. Episodic diarrhea may result ...m a food allergy or from inges-...n of spicy or high-fiber foods or ...ffeine.

Characteristics of diarrheal stool ...ay suggest the underlying cause.

CHECKLIST

Vomitus: Characteristics and causes

When you collect a sample of a pa-tient's vomitus, examine it carefully for clues to the underlying disorder. Here's what vomitus may indicate:
☐ bilious (greenish) vomitus — obstruction below the pylorus, as from a duodenal lesion.
☐ bloody vomitus — upper GI bleeding, as from gastritis or peptic ulcer (if bright red), or from esophageal or gastric varices (if dark red)
☐ brown vomitus with a fecal odor — intestinal obstruction or infarction
☐ coffee-ground vomitus — digested blood from slowly bleeding gastric or duodenal lesion
☐ undigested food in vomitus — gastric outlet obstruction, as from gastric tu-mor or ulcer.

For example, bloody diarrhea may result from bowel inflammation or neoplasm. A bulky, greasy stool points to a fat malabsorption disor-der secondary to gallbladder dis-ease.

Parasitic infection — from recent foreign travel, for instance — can also produce diarrhea. Certain drugs as well as changes in a medication regimen may cause diarrhea. Anti-biotic therapy, for example, may cause pseudomembranous enteroco-litis with accompanying diarrhea.

During rapid assessment, keep in mind that severe diarrhea can lead to fluid and electrolyte imbalances. Such imbalances can precipitate life-threatening cardiac arrhythmias or hypovolemia, calling for immediate intervention.

Constipation. If the patient com-plains of constipation, explore his problem by asking appropriate questions from this list.

• When did the patient first feel constipated? Find out when he had his last bowel movement, and have him describe the stool.

• Does the constipation seem to be getting better or worse, or staying about the same? What, if anything, seems to relieve the constipation? What makes it worse?

• Ask about related symptoms, such as abdominal pain, cramping, distention, or bloating.

• What's the patient's regular pattern of bowel movements? Have him describe the usual size and character of his stools.

• Has he recently changed his eating habits or physical activities? If so, in what way?

• Does he take laxatives or other medications? If so, what does he take, how much, and how often? Has he recently changed medications?

Analyzing the chief complaint. Defined as small, infrequent, or difficult bowel movements, constipation may be a minor annoyance or, less commonly, a sign of a life-threatening disorder such as acute intestinal obstruction. Because normal bowel patterns vary among individuals, constipation must be determined in relation to the patient's normal pattern.

Commonly, constipation occurs when the urge to defecate is suppressed and the muscles associated with bowel movements remain contracted. Because the autonomic nervous system controls bowel movements—by sensing rectal distention from fecal contents and stimulating the external sphincter—any factor that influences the nervous system may cause bowel dysfunction. (See *How constipation can develop.*)

Acute constipation usually has an organic cause, such as an anal or rectal disorder. In a patient over age 45, recent onset of constipation may be an early sign of colorectal cancer. Conversely, chronic constipation typically has a functional cause.

Constipation accompanied by cramping abdominal pain and distention suggests obstipation—extreme, persistent constipation caused by intestinal tract obstruction. If the patient reports pain relieved on elimination, suspect irritable bowel syndrome. Other common causes of constipation include long-term use of laxatives or enemas, other medications, and prolonged immobility.

Changes in voiding patterns. If the patient reports changes in voiding patterns, explore his problem by asking appropriate questions from this list.

• Find out what kind of problem the patient is experiencing. Has he noticed a change in urine amount, color, or odor? Has the size or force of the urine stream, the frequency of urination, or his ability to control or release urine changed?

• When did he first notice the change? Was the onset sudden or gradual? Has the problem occurred before? If so, when and how was it relieved?

• Is the problem constant or intermittent? Does it interfere with his sleep? Does anything relieve or aggravate the problem?

• Ask about related symptoms, such as pain, fever, or bleeding.

• Find out what medications the patient is taking, if any. How much does he take, and how often?

Analyzing the chief complaint. Significant changes in voiding patterns

ow constipation can develop

The chart below lists some possible causes of constipation and describes how constipation develops with each.

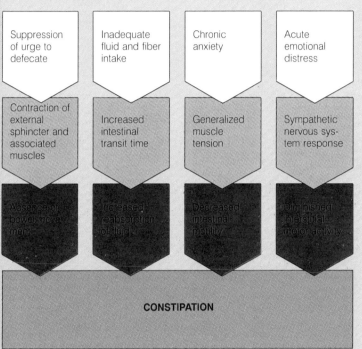

| Suppression of urge to defecate | Inadequate fluid and fiber intake | Chronic anxiety | Acute emotional distress |

| Contraction of external sphincter and associated muscles | Increased intestinal transit time | Generalized muscle tension | Sympathetic nervous system response |

| Absence of bowel movement | Increased reabsorption of fluid | Decreased intestinal motility | Diminished intestinal motor activity |

CONSTIPATION

clude those affecting the volume
ad appearance of urine, the fre-
uency of voiding, and the patient's
ility to control voiding.

Changes in volume considered
nically significant include oliguria,
uria, and polyuria. Defined as
ine output of less than 400 ml in
hours, oliguria is a cardinal sign
renal and urologic disorders. Typ-
ally, this sign occurs abruptly and
ay herald serious hemodynamic inability. Its causes can be classified
prerenal (disorders that decrease
nal blood flow, such as hypovole-

mia), intrarenal (intrinsic renal damage such as acute tubular necrosis),
or postrenal (urinary tract obstruction such as from benign prostatic
hypertrophy).

Anuria, defined as urine output of
less than 75 ml daily, indicates either urinary tract obstruction or
acute renal failure caused by various mechanisms. However, anuria
rarely occurs — even in renal failure.
If you detect anuria, determine
whether urine formation is occurring by assessing the bladder for
distention, and intervene appropri-

ately. Without immediate treatment, anuria can rapidly cause uremia and other complications of urine retention.

A relatively common sign, polyuria is the daily production and excretion of more than 2,500 ml of urine. It's usually reported by the patient as increased voidings, especially occurring at night. Polyuria most commonly results from diabetes insipidus or diabetes mellitus, psychological or neurologic disorders, renal or urologic disorders (such as pyelonephritis or postobstructive uropathy), and use of drugs (such as diuretics). Because the patient with polyuria is at risk for developing hypovolemia, carefully assess his fluid status.

• *Changes in urine appearance* provide important diagnostic clues. A clear, watery appearance may indicate dilute urine, associated with increased volume. A dark amber color may indicate concentrated urine, usually associated with diminished volume.

Brown or bright red urine may contain blood (hematuria). A cardinal sign of renal and urologic disorders, hematuria may be classified by the stage of urination it primarily affects. Bleeding at the start of urination usually indicates a urethral disorder; bleeding at the end of urination, a disorder of the bladder neck, posterior urethra, or prostate. Bleeding throughout urination usually indicates a disorder above the bladder neck.

Although hematuria usually results from renal and urologic disorders, it also may result from certain GI, prostate, vaginal, or coagulation disorders, or from the effects of drugs. Invasive therapy or diagnostic tests that involve instrumentation of the renal and urologic systems may also cause hematuria.

Nonpathologic hematuria may resu from fever and hypercatabolic states. Transient hematuria may also follow strenuous exercise.

Other urine color variations may result from certain medications, such as cyclophosphamide and metyrosine. (See *Evaluating urine appearance.*)

• *Urinary frequency,* or an increase urge to void, commonly results fro decreased bladder capacity and is a cardinal symptom of urinary tract infection. However, it can also stem from other urologic disorders such as benign prostatic hypertrophy an urethral stricture or from neurolog dysfunction such as a spinal cord le sion. Urinary frequency also may b caused by pressure on the bladder from a nearby tumor such as in the prostate or uterus or from organ en largement such as during pregnancy. Even constipation can cause urinary frequency because of the pressure retained stool puts on the bladder.

• *Urinary urgency,* or a sudden con pelling urge to urinate, accompanie by bladder pain, is a classic symptom of urinary tract infection. As in flammation decreases bladder capacity, discomfort results from th accumulation of even small amount of urine. Repeated frequent voiding in an effort to alleviate this discom fort produces little urine output at each voiding. Urgency without blac der pain may point to an upper mo tor neuron lesion that has disrupte bladder control.

• *Urinary hesitancy,* or difficulty starting a urine stream, can result from a urinary tract infection, a pa tial lower urinary tract obstruction a neuromuscular disorder, or use o certain drugs. Occurring at all age and in both sexes, hesitancy is mo common in older men with prostati enlargement. It usually arises grad ually, often going unnoticed until urine retention causes bladder distention and discomfort.

• *Nocturia,* or excessive urination at night, may result from disruption of the normal diurnal pattern of urine concentration or from overstimulation of the nerves and muscles that control urination. Although nocturia usually results from renal and lower urinary tract disorders, it also may result from certain cardiovascular, endocrine, and metabolic disorders. This common sign also can result from drugs that induce diuresis and from ingestion of large quantities of fluids, especially caffeinated beverages or alcohol, at bedtime.

• *Urinary incontinence,* or the uncontrollable passage of urine, most commonly results from benign prostatic hypertrophy, prostatic infection or tumor, bladder cancer or calculi, and neurologic disorders, such as multiple sclerosis, Guillain-Barré syndrome, and spinal cord injury. It also may be the first sign of a urinary tract infection.

A common urologic complaint, incontinence may be transient or permanent and may involve a small or large amount of urine. It can be classified as stress, urge, overflow, or total incontinence. Stress incontinence refers to intermittent urine leakage in response to suddenly increased abdominal pressure — for instance, when a person sneezes or coughs. Urge incontinence is the inability to suppress a sudden urge to urinate. Overflow incontinence refers to dribbling resulting from urine retention. In this case, the full bladder can't contract with enough force to produce a urine stream. Total incontinence is a continuous leakage resulting from the bladder's inability to retain any urine.

Dysuria usually reflects lower urinary tract infection. The patient

Evaluating urine appearance

Carefully examining a patient's urine specimen can give you an important clue to his underlying problem. Here's what the appearance of urine may indicate:

☐ cloudy — infection, inflammation, glomerular nephritis, vegetarian diet
☐ colorless or pale straw color (dilute urine) — excessive fluid intake, anxiety, chronic renal disease, diabetes insipidus, diuretic therapy
☐ dark brown or black — acute glomerulonephritis, drugs such as nitrofurantoin and chlorpromazine
☐ dark yellow or amber (concentrated urine) — low fluid intake, acute febrile disease, vomiting or diarrhea causing large fluid loss
☐ green-brown — bile duct obstruction
☐ orange-red to orange-brown — urobilinuria, drugs such as phenazopyridine, obstructive jaundice (tea-colored urine)
☐ red or red-brown — porphyria, hemorrhage, drugs such as phenazopyridine or sulfobromophthalein.

may report a burning sensation or actual pain on urination. The onset of pain provides clues to its cause. For example, pain just before voiding usually indicates bladder irritation or distention; pain at the start of urination typically results from bladder outlet irritation; and pain at the end of voiding may signal bladder spasms. Pain throughout voiding may indicate acute pyelonephritis, a more serious infection — especially when accompanied by persistent high fever with chills, CVA tenderness, hematuria, or flank pain.

Rectal bleeding. If the patient reports rectal bleeding, explore his problem by asking appropriate

questions from this list.
- When did the patient first notice the rectal bleeding? Did it start suddenly or gradually?
- Is the bleeding constant or intermittent? Does it occur with every bowel movement? Does anything seem to relieve it? Make it worse?
- Have the patient describe the color and consistency of his stools. Do they always look the same, or do they vary?
- Ask about related symptoms, such as abdominal cramps or pain and dizziness.
- Does the patient have a history of hemorrhoids? Also find out about any previous surgery involving the intestines or rectum.
- Ask what medications the patient is taking. Find out how much he takes and how often.

Analyzing the chief complaint. Associated with the passage of bloody stools, rectal bleeding usually indicates GI hemorrhage below the ligament of Treitz, such as from anal fissures, anorectal fistulas, colon cancer, colitis, or hemorrhoids. In many cases, rectal bleeding is the first sign of lower GI tract bleeding. Rectal bleeding preceded by hematemesis also may accompany severe upper GI tract hemorrhage, such as bleeding esophageal varices. Always a significant sign, rectal bleeding may precipitate life-threatening hypovolemia.

Ranging from formed blood-streaked stools to liquid bloody stools that may appear bright red, dark mahogany, or maroon, rectal bleeding typically develops abruptly and is accompanied by abdominal pain.

Although rectal bleeding most commonly results from GI disorders, it also may result from coagulation disorders, such as thrombocytopenia

and disseminated intravascular coagulation; effects of toxins, such as staphylococcal food poisoning and heavy metal poisoning; and certain invasive diagnostic tests, such as colonoscopy.

Abnormal vaginal bleeding. If the patient reports abnormal vaginal bleeding, explore her problem by asking appropriate questions from this list.
- When did the patient first notice the vaginal bleeding? How long has it been occurring?
- Does the bleeding occur during or after intercourse, or spontaneously?
- Ask about related symptoms, such as cramping or passing clots.
- Ask about her menstrual periods. When was her last period and how long did it last? Has the usual duration of the period or the nature of flow changed recently? If flow has been heavier than usual, how many additional tampons or pads has she been using?
- Is the patient pregnant?

Analyzing the chief complaint. Abnormal vaginal bleeding takes three basic forms — menorrhagia, metrorrhagia, and postmenopausal bleeding. Profuse or extended menstrual bleeding, menorrhagia may involve normal flow of increased duration or heavier flow of normal duration. Its most common causes include uterine fibroids and endometriosis. It also may be related to blood disorders such as thrombocytopenia, stress, certain drugs such as anticoagulants and salicylates, and invasive procedures.

Vaginal bleeding occurring irregularly between menstrual periods, metrorrhagia can range from slight staining to frank hemorrhage. Most often, this common sign reflects slight physiologic bleeding from the endometrium during ovulation. In some cases, however, it may be the only indication of an underlying gynecologic disorder, such as an ovarian or uterine tumor. It also can result from stress, drugs, and use of an intrauterine contraceptive device.

Postmenopausal bleeding — bleeding occurring 6 or more months after menopause — is an important sign of gynecologic cancer. It also can result from infection, local pelvic disorders, estrogenic stimulation, and normal physiologic thinning of the vaginal mucosa.

If a pregnant patient reports abnormal vaginal bleeding, notify the doctor. In any patient reporting heavy vaginal bleeding, assess for signs of hypovolemia or shock and intervene as necessary.

Physical assessment

To assess the abdomen, you'll perform the four standard techniques — but not in the usual order. Instead, you'll follow this sequence: inspection, auscultation, percussion, and palpation. This sequence ensures that you don't alter bowel sounds with percussion and palpation before you auscultate them. And percussing before palpating ensures that palpation — especially deep palpation — doesn't alter your percussion findings.

Before assessing your patient's abdomen, check for contraindications to percussion and palpation. Avoid abdominal percussion or palpation on a patient with newly transplanted kidneys or other organs. Also, never palpate the abdomen of a patient who may have appendicitis or a dissecting abdominal aortic aneurysm. Doing so could cause a rupture. And don't perform palpation on a patient who may have polycystic kidneys — you may dislodge a cyst.

Depending on your patient's chief complaint, certain aspects of inspection, auscultation, percussion, and palpation will assume greater priority. Other aspects will become less important or perhaps even unnecessary.

As you perform your assessment, keep in mind the normal findings for the abdomen. (See *Abdomen: Normal findings,* page 138.) With a pregnant patient, remember the normal variations: increased pigmentation of the abdominal midline, purplish striae, and upward displacement of the abdominal organs and the umbilicus.

Preparation. Make sure the patient is in the supine position with his arms at his sides and his head on a pillow to help relax the abdominal muscles. If you're examining a pregnant patient, vary the assessment position depending on the stage of pregnancy. For example, in the final weeks, the patient may find the supine position uncomfortable because it can impair respiratory excursion and blood flow. To enhance comfort, have her lie on her side or assume the semi-Fowler's position.

Mentally divide the abdomen into quadrants or regions for assessment. (See *Reviewing abdominal quadrants and regions,* pages 140 and 141.) Systematically assess all areas, if time and the patient's condition permit, concluding with the symptomatic area. Otherwise, you may elicit pain in the symptomatic area, causing the muscles in other areas to tighten. This would interfere with further assessment.

Inspection. Examine the patient's entire abdomen, observing overall contour, color, and skin integrity. Look for any rashes, scars, or incisions from past surgeries. Observe

CHECKLIST

Abdomen: Normal findings

Inspection
Normal findings include:
- [ ] skin free from vascular lesions, jaundice, surgical scars, and rashes
- [ ] faint venous patterns (except in thin patients)
- [ ] flat, round, or scaphoid abdominal contour
- [ ] symmetrical abdomen
- [ ] umbilicus positioned midway between the xiphoid process and the symphysis pubis, with a flat or concave hemisphere
- [ ] no variations in the color of the patient's skin
- [ ] no apparent bulges
- [ ] abdominal movement apparent with respiration
- [ ] pink or silver-white striae from pregnancy or weight loss.

Auscultation
Normal findings include:
- [ ] high-pitched, gurgling bowel sounds, every 5 to 15 seconds through the diaphragm of the stethoscope
- [ ] vascular sounds through the bell of the stethoscope
- [ ] venous hum over the inferior vena cava
- [ ] no bruits, murmurs, friction rubs, or other venous hums.

Percussion
Normal findings include:
- [ ] tympany predominantly over hollow organs including the stomach, intestines, bladder, abdominal aorta, and gallbladder
- [ ] dullness over solid masses including the liver, spleen, pancreas, kidneys, uterus, and a full bladder.

Palpation
Normal findings include:
- [ ] no tenderness or masses
- [ ] abdominal musculature free from tenderness and rigidity
- [ ] no guarding, rebound tenderness, distention, or ascites
- [ ] unpalpable liver except in children (If palpable, liver edge is regular, sharp, and nontender and felt no more than ¾" [2 cm] below the right costal margin.)
- [ ] unpalpable spleen
- [ ] unpalpable kidneys except in thin patients or those with a flaccid abdominal wall. (Right kidney felt more commonly than the left. When palpable, kidney is solid and firm.)

the umbilicus for protrusions or discoloration.

Note any visible abdominal asymmetry, masses, pulsations, or peristalsis. You can detect masses — especially hepatic and splenic — more easily by inspecting the areas while the patient takes a deep breath and holds it. This forces the diaphragm downward, increasing intra-abdominal pressure and reducing the size of the abdominal cavity.

Although not commonly considered part of abdominal assessment, inspecting the external genitalia may be appropriate in some patients. Remember, many problems associated with the genitalia are reflected as abdominal complaints. Inspect the pubis, urinary meatus, labia, and vaginal opening in females, and the penis and scrotum in males. Note any redness, irritation, inflammation, drainage, or lesions that might indicate an infectious process. Also look for frank bleeding, noting the amount, character, and source. If you suspect a urinary problem, obtain a urine specimen and assess its color, odor, and clarity.

Finally, examine the rectal area for redness, irritation, or hemorrhoids.

Interpreting your findings. A concave abdomen may be associated with cachexia. A protruding abdomen may result from obesity, as well as from ascites, bladder distention, gaseous distention, or organomegaly.

Visible skin abnormalities often provide valuable clues to abdominal problems. Bulging around old scars may indicate an incisional hernia. Striae commonly result from obesity or pregnancy but also may result from an abdominal tumor or other disorder. Newly developed striae usually appear pink or blue; older striae appear white or silver. Tense, glistening skin may indicate ascites. Dilated, tortuous superficial abdominal veins may point to inferior vena cava obstruction or may accompany other vascular signs associated with liver disease.

An everted umbilicus is normal in some patients. In others, it may signal increased intra-abdominal pressure from ascites or a large mass. An everted umbilicus also can result from an umbilical hernia. To quickly check for an umbilical or other abdominal hernia, have the patient raise his head and shoulders while remaining supine. A true hernia may protrude during this maneuver.

A bluish tinge around the umbilicus (also known as Cullen's sign) may point to intra-abdominal bleeding. Massive ecchymoses on the abdomen and flanks may indicate hemorrhagic pancreatitis or a strangulated bowel.

Localized swelling or asymmetry may signal hernias or organomeg-

aly. Strong visible peristaltic waves commonly indicate intestinal obstruction; report this finding immediately. Abdominal aortic pulsations may become more pronounced and obvious from increased intra-abdominal pressure, as from a tumor or ascites. Abnormal abdominal pulsations, along with vital sign and skin color changes consistent with shock, are clues to a dissecting abdominal aortic aneurysm. If you suspect an aneurysm, notify the doctor immediately.

Auscultation. Next, auscultate the abdomen to detect sounds that provide information on bowel motility and the condition of abdominal vessels and organs.

To auscultate bowel sounds, which result from air and fluid movement through the bowel, press the diaphragm of the stethoscope against the abdomen and listen carefully. Auscultate the quadrants systematically. In a routine complete assessment, you'd auscultate for a full 5 minutes before determining that bowel sounds are absent. In a rapid assessment, however, cut this time short. If you can't hear bowel sounds within 2 minutes, suspect a serious problem. Even if subsequent palpation stimulates peristalsis, still report a long silence in that quadrant. Be sure to describe bowel sounds accurately — for example, as quiet or loud gurgles, occasional gurgles, fine tinkles, or loud tinkles.

Next, lightly apply the bell of the stethoscope to each quadrant. Listen for vascular sounds, such as bruits and venous hums, and for friction rubs.

Interpreting your findings. Abdominal auscultation may reveal abnormal bowel sounds, bruits, venous

Reviewing abdominal quadrants and regions

For assessment purposes, the abdomen is commonly divided into quadrants with the umbilicus as the center point. As an alternative, you can divide the abdomen into nine regions.

ABDOMINAL QUADRANTS

Right upper quadrant (RUQ)
Liver and gallbladder
Pylorus
Duodenum
Head of pancreas
Hepatic flexure of colon
Right kidney
Portions of ascending and transverse colon

Left upper quadrant (LUQ)
Left liver lobe
Stomach
Left kidney
Body of pancreas
Spleen
Splenic flexure of colon
Portions of transverse and descending colon

Right lower quadrant (RLQ)
Cecum
Appendix
Portions of ascending colon, abdominal aorta, vena cava, bladder, and rectum
Right ureter

Left lower quadrant (LLQ)
Sigmoid colon
Portions of descending colon, abdominal aorta, small intestine, vena cava, bladder, and rectum
Left ureter

NINE ABDOMINAL REGIONS

Right hypochondriac
Right liver lobe
Gallbladder
Portion of right kidney

Epigastric
Pyloric end of stomach
Duodenum
Pancreas
Portion of liver

Left hypochondriac
Stomach
Tail of pancreas
Spleen
Splenic flexure of colon
Portion of left kidney

Right lumbar
Ascending colon
Portion of right kidney
Portions of duodenum and jejunum
Portion of right ureter

Umbilical or middle epigastric
Abdominal aorta
Vena cava
Lower part of duodenum
Jejunum and ileum
Ureters

Left lumbar
Descending colon
Portion of left kidney
Portions of jejunum and ileum
Portion of left ureter

Right inguinal
Cecum
Appendix
Lower end of ileum

Suprapubic or hypogastric
Ileum
Bladder
Rectum
Portions of ureters, vena cava, and abdominal aorta

Left inguinal
Sigmoid colon

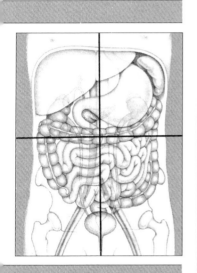

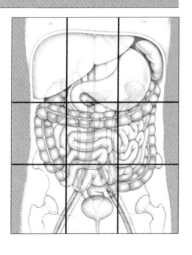

hums, or friction rubs. (See *Understanding abnormal abdominal sounds,* page 142, for more information.)

Percussion. An important technique in rapid assessment, percussion can help you quickly identify areas of abdominal tenderness, gaseous distention, ascites, or solid masses. Systematically percuss in all abdominal areas, keeping the approximate location of underlying organs in mind as you progress. Concentrate on areas of obvious enlargement or pain. When assessing a tender abdomen, have the patient cough, then lightly percuss where the cough produced the pain. This can help localize the involved area. As you percuss, note areas of dullness, tympany, and flatness, as well as any patient complaints of tenderness.

You won't routinely percuss the liver in a rapid assessment. But when you suspect or know that the patient has a liver disease, you may percuss to estimate liver size. (See *Percussing the liver,* page 143, for a description of this technique.) With a normal liver, you'll hear dullness for 2½" to 5" (6 to 12 cm) along the right midclavicular line and 1½" to 3" (4 to 8 cm) along the midsternal line. With a normal spleen, you'll hear dullness between the 6th and 11th ribs on the midaxillary line.

Interpreting your findings. Abnormal percussion findings commonly occur in patients with abdominal distention from gas accumulation, ascites, or masses. Extremely high-pitched tympanic notes may indicate gaseous bowel distention. Ascites may produce dull percussion notes over the flanks. A solid tumor in the lower abdomen will cause dullness.

Abnormal liver size may point to

Understanding abnormal abdominal sounds

SOUND AND DESCRIPTION	LOCATION	POSSIBLE CAUSE
Abnormal bowel sounds		
• Hyperactive sounds (unrelated to hunger)	• Any quadrant	• Diarrhea or early intestinal obstruction
• Hypoactive, then absent sounds	• Any quadrant	• Paralytic ileus or peritonitis
• High-pitched tinkling sounds	• Any quadrant	• Intestinal fluid and air under tension in a dilated bowel
• High-pitched rushing sounds coinciding with abdominal cramps	• Any quadrant	• Intestinal obstruction
Systolic bruits Vascular blowing sounds resembling cardiac murmurs	• Over abdominal aorta • Over renal artery • Over iliac artery	• Partial arterial obstruction or turbulent blood flow • Renal artery stenosis • Hepatomegaly
Venous hum Continuous, medium-pitched tone created by blood flow in a large, engorged vascular organ such as the liver	• Epigastric and umbilical regions	• Increased collateral circulation between portal and systemic venous systems, as in hepatic cirrhosis
Friction rub Harsh, grating sound resembling two pieces of sandpaper rubbing together	• Over liver	• Inflammation of the peritoneal surface of liver, as from a tumor

underlying disease. For instance, a patient with hepatitis may have an enlarged, tender liver; a patient with cirrhosis, a small, hard liver.

Palpation. In rapid assessment, you'll palpate primarily to detect areas of pain and tenderness, guarding, rebound tenderness, and CVA tenderness, using light and deep palpation as necessary. Abdominal palpation also provides useful clues about the character of the abdominal wall, the presence and nature of any abdominal masses, and the size, condition, and consistency of abdominal organs.

Light palpation. Use light palpation to detect tenderness, areas of mus-

cle spasm or rigidity, and superficial masses. With the pads of your fingers, press gently into the patient's abdomen to a depth of about ½" (1 cm). To aid palpation for superficial masses in the abdominal wall, have the patient raise his head and shoulders, which will tighten the abdominal muscles. A deep mass will be obscured by muscular tension, but an abdominal wall mass will remain palpable. This technique also may help you determine whether pain originates from the abdominal muscles or from deeper structures.

If you detect tenderness, assess for involuntary guarding, or abdominal rigidity. As the patient exhales, palpate the abdominal rectus muscles. Normally, they should soften and relax on exhalation; note abnormal muscle tension or inflexibility. Involuntary guarding points to peritoneal irritation, possibly associated with a condition such as acute appendicitis, acute cholecystitis, pelvic inflammatory disease, diverticulitis, or ruptured ectopic pregnancy. In generalized peritonitis, rigidity is severe and diffuse, commonly described as a "board-like" abdomen.

A tense or ticklish patient may exhibit voluntary guarding. Help this patient relax by instructing him to breathe deeply and slowly, inhaling through his nose and exhaling through his mouth.

If a patient complains of abdominal pain, check for rebound tenderness. Because this maneuver can be painful, perform it near the end of your abdominal assessment. Press your fingertips into the site where the patient reports pain or tenderness. As you quickly release the pressure, the abdominal tissue will rebound. If the patient reports pain as the tissue springs back, you've elicited rebound tenderness. (See *Eliciting rebound tenderness*, page 144.)

Deep palpation. Next, if time permits, perform deep abdominal palpation to detect deep tenderness or masses and to evaluate organ size. Using the pads of your fingers, press gently but steadily into the abdominal wall to a depth of about 1½" (4 cm). If you feel a mass, note its size, shape, consistency, and location. If the patient complains of pain or tenderness, note its location and whether it's generalized or localized. Also note any guarding the patient exhibits during deep palpation. You may feel a tensing of a small or large area of abdominal musculature directly below your fingers.

Percussing the liver

In certain cases, you may percuss a patient's liver to estimate its size and position. Be sure to instruct him to hold his breath as you percuss. This keeps the liver from moving up and down during your assessment.

With the patient in the supine position, start percussing on the right midclavicular line (MCL) about 2 fingerbreadths below the nipple. Because you'll be over lung tissue, you'll hear a resonant percussion sound. As you move down the MCL, the sound will become dull, indicating the liver's upper border. Usually, you'll hear the change somewhere between the fifth and seventh intercostal spaces, as shown. Mark the location with a water-soluble marker.

Locating the liver's upper border

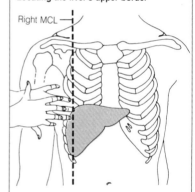

Right MCL

To find the liver's lower border, start percussing on the right MCL about 3 fingerbreadths below the level of the umbilicus and move upward. When the sound changes from tympany to dullness, you've located the lower border of the liver. Mark that location, too.

Measure the distance between the upper and lower borders to determine liver size. The normal liver span on the MCL is between 2½" and 5" (6 and 12 cm).

Eliciting rebound tenderness

To elicit rebound tenderness, a reliable sign of peritoneal irritation, press your fingertips deeply and gently into the area on the patient's abdomen where he reports pain or tenderness.

Quickly withdraw your fingertips. If the patient complains of pain at the site when the tissue springs back, you've elicited rebound tenderness.

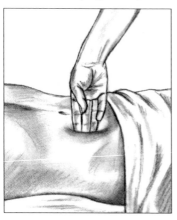

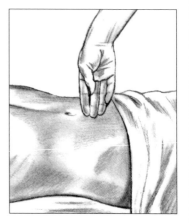

If a patient is suspected of having cholecystitis, palpate the right subcostal area while he takes a deep breath. A patient with gallbladder distention from cholecystitis will stop inhaling to guard against the pain produced by palpation — a finding known as Murphy's sign.

Palpate the patient's bladder, noting any distention or masses. If the patient reports pain during palpation, proceed carefully — suprapubic pain or tenderness is commonly associated with cystitis. You may palpate a full bladder as high as the umbilicus and a greatly distended bladder (as from urine retention) above the umbilicus. In a patient with chronic urine retention, the bladder walls will feel flabby on palpation.

Palpate the CVA for tenderness, which may indicate a renal problem. Locate the CVA by identifying the junction between the twelfth rib and the spinal column. (See *Identifying the costovertebral angle.*) Some examiners percuss this area with a fist to elicit tenderness. However, if your patient is an older woman, palpate gently to avoid causing a spinal compression fracture. If the patient complains of tenderness or pain on CVA palpation, palpate several other areas on his back. If palpation elicits pain in those areas, suspect muscular origin. If not, suspect renal involvement. Common causes of CVA tenderness include pyelonephritis, renal infection, calculi, hydronephrosis, and glomerulonephritis.

Further assessment. Because abdominal assessment findings can reflect problems in organs and structures outside the abdomen, you may need to assess other body regions. For example, pulmonary problems such as pneumonia or pulmonary edema can cause severe upper abdominal pain and rigidity.

If a patient with nausea also reports tinnitus or hearing loss, suspect an inner ear disturbance. In a patient with vomiting and an accompanying severe headache, assess for a neurologic disturbance.

If a patient's kidney function is impaired, assess for edema and other signs of fluid imbalance. Also, auscultate the lungs for signs of pulmonary edema and inspect his neck for jugular vein distention.

Once you've obtained the necessary information about the patient's chief complaint and completed your physical assessment, you'll begin to formulate a diagnostic impression. (See *Abdomen: Interpreting your findings,* pages 146 to 148.)

Pediatric considerations

When you rapidly assess the abdomen of an infant or child, you'll follow many of the same steps you'd take for an adult. As appropriate, expect to modify your technique to accommodate developmental differences. Begin by positioning the patient, according to his age and level of cooperation. An older child may lie supine on the examining table, but you may need to place a young child or infant across a parent's lap.

General observations. When observing a pediatric patient, note the position of his ears. In children, ears set low or at an unusual angle often accompany urinary tract anomalies.

Inspection. Observing abdominal

Identifying the costovertebral angle

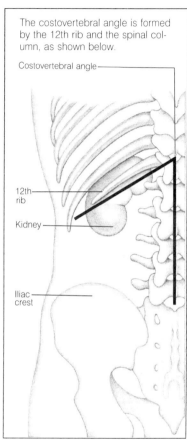

The costovertebral angle is formed by the 12th rib and the spinal column, as shown below.

Costovertebral angle

12th rib

Kidney

Iliac crest

contour in a child may provide the first clues to a possible abdominal disorder. In a child under age 4, mild abdominal distention (a "pot belly") when standing or sitting is a normal finding. In a child age 4 to 13, however, distention is normal only with the child standing. Extreme distention may result from enlargement of the viscera, ascites, a neoplasm, abdominal wall defects,

(Text continues on page 148.)

DIAGNOSTIC IMPRESSION

Abdomen: Interpreting your findings

After you assess the patient, a group of findings may lead you to suspect a particular disorder. The chart below shows you some common groups of findings for the chief complaints of the abdomen, along with the appropriate nursing diagnostic categories and probable causes.

CHIEF COMPLAINT AND FINDINGS	NURSING DIAGNOSTIC CATEGORIES	PROBABLE CAUSE
Abdominal pain		
• Gnawing, burning, and steady pain, occurring high in the midepigastrium or slightly off center; typical onset 2 to 4 hours after meals, with occasional nocturnal awakening; temporarily relieved by ingestion of food or antacids • Abdominal tenderness on palpation • Changes in bowel habits • Melena (black, tarry stools) • Nausea • Vomiting, with possible hematemesis	• Altered nutrition: More than body requirements • Constipation • Diarrhea • Pain • Sleep pattern disturbance	Duodenal ulcer
• Severe, colicky abdominal pain, traveling from costovertebral angle to flank, suprapubic region, and external genitalia • Abdominal distention • Concentrated urine • Fever and chills • Hematuria • Vomiting	• Pain • Potential for infection	Renal colic
• Mild pain occurring in the left lower quadrant and becoming sharp and severe on sudden standing or stooping • Abdominal distention • Mild nausea and vomiting • Occasional menstrual irregularities • Palpable cyst (on bimanual palpation) • Slight fever	• Altered sexuality patterns • Pain • Potential for fluid volume deficit	Functional ovarian cysts
Diarrhea		
• Abdominal tenderness • Anorexia • Cramping and right lower quadrant pain • Emotional stress • Hyperactive bowel sounds • Nausea • Palpable mass in right lower quadrant • Weakness • Weight loss	• Altered nutrition: Less than body requirements • Pain • Potential for fluid volume deficit	Crohn's disease

DIAGNOSTIC IMPRESSION

Abdomen: Interpreting your findings *(continued)*

CHIEF COMPLAINT AND FINDINGS	NURSING DIAGNOSTIC CATEGORIES	PROBABLE CAUSE
Nausea and vomiting		
• Altered sense of taste and smell • Anorexia • Arthralgia • Coryza • Cough • Fatigue • Fever • Headache • Loss of desire to drink alcohol or smoke • Malaise • Myalgia • Palpable enlarged liver • Photophobia	• Altered nutrition: Less than body requirements • Fatigue • Pain • Potential for fluid volume deficit • Sensory-perceptual alterations	Viral hepatitis (preicteric phase)
• Anorexia • Irregular pulse • Malaise • Tremor • Weakness	• Altered nutrition: Less than body requirements • Fatigue • Self-care deficit	Electrolyte imbalance
Constipation		
• Dull, generalized abdominal discomfort described as feeling of fullness • Emotional stress • Hyperactive bowel sounds • Intermittent or alternating diarrhea • Nausea without vomiting • No referred rebound tenderness • Scybalous stools, with visible mucus • Soft, slightly distended abdomen	• Pain	Irritable bowel syndrome
• Abdominal discomfort • Excessive antacid consumption • Normal physical assessment findings • Recent emotional stress • Sedentary life-style	• Anxiety • Constipation • Knowledge deficit • Pain	Drug-induced constipation
Urinary frequency		
• Burning sensation on urination • Fever • Inflamed perineal area • Low back or flank pain • Nocturia • Suprapubic pain on palpation • Urinary urgency	• Altered urinary elimination patterns • Pain • Sleep pattern disturbance • Urge incontinence	Cystitis

(continued)

DIAGNOSTIC IMPRESSION

Abdomen: Interpreting your findings *(continued)*

CHIEF COMPLAINT AND FINDINGS	NURSING DIAGNOSTIC CATEGORIES	PROBABLE CAUSE
Urinary hesitancy		
• Bladder distention • Feeling of incomplete voiding • Frequent urination • Nocturia • Reduced force of urine stream	• Altered urinary elimination patterns • Anxiety • Fluid volume excess • Knowledge deficit • Potential for body image disturbance	Benign prostatic hypertrophy
Rectal bleeding		
• Bleeding and pain on defecation • External hemorrhoids • Pain on movement • Rectal itching	• Impaired physical mobility • Pain	Rectal hemorrhoids
• Slightly to grossly bloody stools • Chronic liver disease • Hypotension • Mild to severe hematemesis • Tachycardia	• Altered tissue perfusion • Anxiety • Fear • Fluid volume deficit	Esophageal varices
Vaginal bleeding		
• Slight spotting • Unilateral pelvic pain possibly increasing to sharp lower abdominal pain	• Anticipatory grieving • Anxiety • Fear • Potential for ineffective coping	Ectopic pregnancy
• Pink discharge increasing to frank bleeding • Increasingly intense abdominal cramps • Positive pregnancy test	• Anticipatory grieving • Anxiety • Fear • Potential for ineffective coping	Spontaneous abortion
• Pain • Uterine enlargement • Weight loss	• Anxiety • Pain • Potential for body image disturbance	Uterine cancer

or starvation. A depressed or concave abdomen may point to diaphragmatic hernia, especially when accompanied by localized swelling.

Note any scars or visible abdominal vascularity. Normally, an infant's superficial veins are readily visible.

During abdominal inspection, remember that a young child's respiratory movements are primarily abdominal; costal movements may indicate peritonitis, intestinal obstruction, or ascites. The transition from abdominal to costal respirations occurs gradually; in most cases, a child breathes abdominally until age 6 or 7.

Although peristaltic waves normally are visible in an infant, visible left-to-right peristaltic waves commonly indicate intestinal obstruction. Right-to-left peristaltic waves commonly point to pyloric stenosis. Other possible causes include bowel malrotation, duodenal ulcer, and duodenal stenosis.

For the best view of an umbilical hernia, wait until the child cries. This increases intra-abdominal pressure and makes herniation more visible.

Auscultation. Perform abdominal auscultation on a child as you would on an adult. Common abnormal findings in children include an abdominal murmur, possibly indicating coarctation of the aorta; a venous hum, suggesting portal hypertension; and a double "pistol shot" sound in the femoral artery, which may signal aortic insufficiency.

Percussion. When percussing an infant's or young child's abdomen, you may hear more tympanic sounds than in an older child or an adult. This normal finding is caused by increased air in the stomach—a result of swallowing air during feeding and crying.

Although you usually can palpate a child's liver rather easily, use percussion to determine liver size. Follow the same procedure as for an adult.

Palpation. You may find abdominal palpation in a child easier than in an

adult because a child's abdominal wall is less well-developed. Tension or ticklishness, however, can hinder accurate palpation. To minimize ticklishness—and to give the child some sense of control over the situation—palpate the abdomen with the child's hand over your own.

If you observe an upper abdominal mass, don't palpate the area. If the mass is a nephroblastoma (Wilm's tumor), palpation could increase the spread of the tumor cell.

Geriatric considerations

You'll use the same assessment techniques and sequence for an elderly patient as you would for any adult patient. Your findings may differ, however, because of normal age-related changes that typically diminish abdominal symptoms. For example, an elderly patient with acute appendicitis may complain only of weakness and anorexia; fever may be less pronounced and muscle guarding may be diminished or absent. So be sure to note even subtle signs and symptoms, and monitor closely for minor changes in baseline findings.

History. Carefully assess bowel habits and function. Decreased tissue perfusion may result from vascular changes, increasing the risk of intestinal ischemia.

In elderly men, changes in voiding patterns should alert you to a possible prostate problem, such as benign prostatic hypertrophy or prostatic cancer. Reduced abdominal muscle tone can interfere with complete bladder emptying, possibly leading to urine retention. Neurologic changes may impair a patient's ability to recognize the urge to void, causing loss of bladder control. This can lead to more serious urinary dysfunction.

Inspection. Before inspecting the abdomen, position the elderly patient as his physical condition permits. For example, an elderly patient with orthopnea may not be able to recline comfortably. Choose a position that he can tolerate and that provides you with good access to the abdomen.

Palpation. With aging, the abdominal wall typically thins from muscle wasting and loss of fibroconnective tissue, and abdominal muscle tone relaxes. For these reasons, abdominal palpation may be easier and the results more accurate in an elderly patient. During assessment, keep in mind that abdominal rigidity is less common and abdominal distention more common in elderly patients. Also remember that an elderly patient is more likely to be taking medications that can affect abdominal assessment results.

Suggested readings

Bates, B., and Hoeckelman, R. *Guide to Physical Examination & History Taking,* 4th ed. Philadelphia: J.B. Lippincott, 1987.

Becker, K., and Stevens, S. "Performing In-Depth Abdominal Assessment," *Nursing88* 18(6):59-63, June 1988.

Lanros, N.E. *Assessment and Intervention in Emergency Nursing,* 3rd ed. Norwalk, Conn.: Appleton & Lange, 1988.

Metzgar, E.D., and Stinger, K.A. *Health Assessment: A Study and Learning Tool.* Springhouse Notes. Springhouse, Pa.: Springhouse Corp., 1988.

Morton, P.G. *Health Assessment in Nursing.* Springhouse, Pa.: Springhouse Corp., 1989.

Munn, N. "Diagnosis: Acute Abdomen," *Nursing88* 18(9):34-42, September 1988.

Swartz, M.H. *Textbook of Physical Diagnosis: History and Examination.* Philadelphia: W.B. Saunders Co., 1989.

7

ASSESSMENT OF THE EXTREMITIES

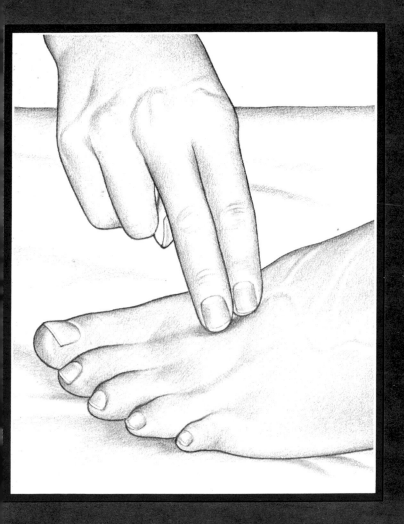

When a patient complains of an arm or a leg problem, you usually don't have a life-threatening situation. But at times you may. A severe injury can lead to blood loss and shock. And a muscle spasm may be the first sign of hypocalcemic tetany.

Typically, your patient's chief complaint will indicate a problem in the bone, muscle, soft-tissue, or neurologic or vascular systems. Or it may signal a disorder in another area—the brain, for instance. To investigate the source of the complaint, you must perform a rapid, systematic assessment.

This chapter reviews the techniques you'll use to rapidly assess the arms and legs of adults. It covers the general observations you'll make and spells out critical questions you'll ask your patient based on his chief complaint. Following the history questions, you'll find an explanation of the physical assessment techniques you'll use. The chapter also covers special considerations for assessing pediatric and elderly patients. And finally, it helps you pull your findings together to develop a diagnostic impression of your patient's problem.

Remember that depending on your findings, you may have to interrupt your assessment of an extremity to examine another part of the body. Or you may need to stop your assessment to provide emergency intervention.

Arms and legs

You'll perform a rapid assessment if your patient complains of a problem in his arm or leg or if you suspect he's injured a limb. Your findings may indicate a range of problems—from a local injury, such as a sprain or fracture, to a systemic problem, such as rheumatoid arthritis. Begin your assessment by making some general observations and taking the patient's vital signs. (See *Reviewing arm and leg structures*, pages 154 and 155.)

General observations

Your general observations of the patient include checking his level of consciousness, his overall appearance, and his skin color.

Level of consciousness. Note whether the patient seems anxious or restless. You may see these signs of shock if the patient has a significant blood loss from a limb injury.

Overall appearance. Observe your patient's overall appearance, including his posture. Note any obvious injuries or deformities of the limbs. Look for muscle atrophy and note whether the limbs are symmetrical.

Skin color. Note any changes in skin color, such as pallor or mottling, which may indicate peripheral hypoperfusion and shock. Depending on the patient's normal skin color, pallor may be difficult to see. In a light-skinned patient, it may be just a subtle lightening of the skin. With a dark-skinned patient, you may need to check his nail beds.

Increased redness, accompanied by heat, may indicate infection or inflammation. Obvious discoloration—such as petechiae, bruising, or ecchymoses—or breaks in skin integrity indicate injury. Also look for lesions, visible masses, and areas of swelling or bleeding.

Vital signs

Take your patient's vital signs and

compare them with baseline measurements. His pulse rate and blood pressure will give you a good indication of blood flow in the limbs.

A fall in systolic blood pressure to 80 mm Hg — or 30 mm Hg less than the patient's baseline — accompanied by a narrowing pulse pressure and a rapid, weak, and, in many cases, irregular pulse may indicate hypovolemic shock.

Unless you suspect infection, you won't need to take a patient's temperature.

History

Obtain a quick history of the patient's chief complaint. The most common chief complaints involving the limbs include pain, swelling, skin color changes, paresthesia, muscle spasm, and changes in mobility or function.

Pain. If your patient complains of pain, explore his problem by asking appropriate questions from this list.
• When did his pain begin? Did it start suddenly or gradually?
• Where is the pain? Is it generalized or localized, constant or intermittent? Ask him to describe it.
• How severe is it? How often does he feel it? How long does it last?
• Is the pain getting better, worse, or staying the same? Is it worse in the morning or at night? Ask what makes it worse and what relieves it.
• Is the pain associated with certain positions, movements, or actions?
• Does he have numbness or tingling? Has he noticed a change in the color or size of the affected limb? Does he have pain anywhere else? If so, where?
• Has he experienced recent trauma or injury to the area where he has the pain?
• Has he had the pain before? When?

Analyzing the chief complaint. The patient may complain of local pain or of pain affecting the entire limb; it may be sudden or gradual, constant or intermittent, sharp or dull, burning or numbing, shooting or penetrating.

If the patient has a fresh fracture, the pain will be intense at the fracture site, worsening with movement. Pain may radiate from the injury site through the limb. Severe pain in a fractured limb after a cast has been applied may indicate limb-threatening compartment syndrome.

If the patient complains of progressive pain, he may have a muscle or tendon that's torn or strained. If he complains of intense, localized pain that's aggravated by movement and relieved by rest, the tendon may be inflamed. Pain after unusual or prolonged exercise that tends to subside with rest may have a muscular origin. Pain near a joint that's aggravated by movement and weight bearing and alleviated by rest probably originates in the joint. If your patient complains of a deep, boring, intense pain that gets worse at night and with weight bearing — and that isn't related to movement — it probably originates in a bone. Pain in an arm or leg may also be referred from another area.
• *Arm pain.* This pain can result from a musculoskeletal problem — muscle strain, sprain, fracture, or a disorder such as osteomyelitis. Muscular pain may result from polymyalgia rheumatica, a collagen disorder. Neurovascular disorders, such as cervical nerve root compression, or cardiovascular disorders, such as myocardial infarction, can also trigger arm pain. Remember, your patient may have trouble describing diffuse arm pain, especially if it isn't associated with an injury.

(Text continues on page 156.)

ANATOMY

Reviewing arm and leg structures

These two illustrations show the major muscles and bones of the arms and legs.

ANTERIOR VIEW

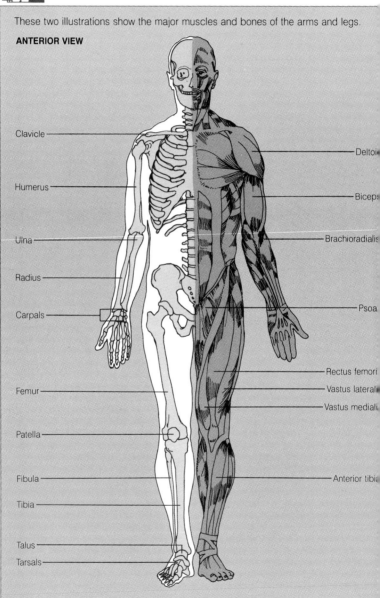

Clavicle

Humerus

Ulna

Radius

Carpals

Femur

Patella

Fibula

Tibia

Talus

Tarsals

Deltoid

Biceps

Brachioradialis

Psoas

Rectus femoris

Vastus lateralis

Vastus medialis

Anterior tibial

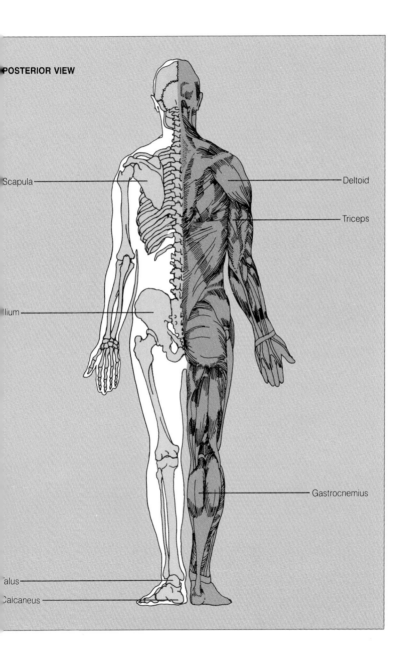

POSTERIOR VIEW

Scapula

Deltoid

Triceps

Ilium

Gastrocnemius

Talus

Calcaneus

Reviewing causes of local pain

Local arm or leg pain may result from these disorders. With some, the pain radiates from other areas; with others, the pain originates in the limb.

Shoulder pain
☐ Acromioclavicular separation
☐ Acute pancreatitis
☐ Adhesive capsulitis (frozen shoulder)
☐ Angina pectoris
☐ Arthritis
☐ Bursitis
☐ Cholecystitis/cholelithiasis
☐ Clavicle fracture
☐ Diaphragmatic pleurisy
☐ Dislocation
☐ Dissecting aortic aneurysm
☐ Gastritis
☐ Humeral neck fracture
☐ Infection
☐ Pancoast's syndrome
☐ Perforated ulcer
☐ Pneumothorax
☐ Ruptured spleen (left shoulder)
☐ Shoulder-hand syndrome
☐ Subphrenic abscess
☐ Tendinitis

Elbow pain
☐ Arthritis
☐ Bursitis
☐ Dislocation
☐ Fracture
☐ Lateral epicondylitis (tennis elbow)
☐ Tendinitis

Wrist pain
☐ Arthritis
☐ Carpal tunnel syndrome
☐ Fracture
☐ Ganglion

☐ Sprain or strain
☐ Tenosynovitis (de Quervain's disease)

Hand pain
☐ Arthritis
☐ Buerger's disease
☐ Carpal tunnel syndrome
☐ Dupuytren's contracture
☐ Elbow tunnel syndrome
☐ Fracture
☐ Ganglion
☐ Infection
☐ Occlusive vascular disease
☐ Radiculopathy
☐ Raynaud's disease
☐ Reflex sympathetic dystrophy
☐ Shoulder-hand syndrome
☐ Sprain or strain
☐ Thoracic outlet syndrome
☐ Trigger finger

Hip pain
☐ Arthritis
☐ Avascular necrosis
☐ Bursitis
☐ Dislocation
☐ Fracture
☐ Sepsis
☐ Tumor

Knee pain
☐ Arthritis
☐ Bursitis
☐ Chondromalacia
☐ Contusion
☐ Cruciate ligament injury

• *Leg pain.* This pain often indicates a musculoskeletal disorder; however, it may also result from a vascular problem, such as thrombophlebitis or occlusive vascular disease, or from a neurologic disorder, such as sciatica, spinal stenosis, or a herniated disk. (See *Reviewing causes of local pain.*)

Pain from occlusive vascular disease usually causes continuous foot and leg cramps and worsens with

Dislocation
Fracture
Meniscal injury
Osteochondritis dissecans
Phlebitis
Popliteal cyst
Radiculopathy
Ruptured extensor mechanism
Sprain

Ankle pain
Achilles tendon contracture
Arthritis
Dislocation
Fracture
Sprain
Tenosynovitis

Foot pain
Arthritis
Bunion
Callus or corn
Dislocation
Flat foot
Fracture
Gout
Hallux rigidus
Hammertoe
Ingrown toenail
Köhler's bone disease
Morton's neuroma
Occlusive vascular disease
Plantar fasciitis
Plantar wart
Radiculopathy
Tabes dorsalis
Tarsal tunnel syndrome

walking. The patient may report increased pain at night and complain of cold feet and intolerance to cold. He may have swelling in the ankle and lower leg, along with decreased or absent pulses and decreased cap-

illary refill time. If a patient with underlying vascular insufficiency suddenly experiences severe pain, suspect acute deterioration, which may necessitate a graft or amputation.

Leg pain may affect a patient's locomotion or limit his weight bearing. Sciatica, for instance, produces tingling, aching, or shooting pain that radiates down the back of the leg. Activity usually exacerbates the pain, and rest relieves it. You may also find that the patient has difficulty standing or limps to avoid increasing the pain.

Swelling. If your patient complains of swelling, explore his problem by asking appropriate questions from this list.
• When did the swelling start? How long has the limb been swollen? Did the swelling develop gradually or suddenly? Is the swelling bilateral?
• Ask what makes the swelling worse and what, if anything, makes it better. Does the swelling increase with activity?
• Does the patient have any pain, numbness, or tingling with the swelling? Does his clothing leave a mark or indentation on the swollen area?
• Has he recently injured the limb or had surgery on it? If so, have him describe the injury or surgery.
• Does he have a history of heart problems? If so, what treatment is he receiving?

Analyzing the chief complaint. Swelling, the result of excess accumulated fluid in the interstitial spaces of the arm or leg, can occur gradually or suddenly. It may be unilateral or bilateral, slight or dramatic, pitting or nonpitting.

Localized joint swelling may indicate synovial inflammation or increased synovial fluid. Joint swelling after an injury may result from blood within the capsule. Slow joint swelling may be caused by increasing synovial fluid. Swelling from pus within the joint can occur quickly or slowly. Generalized swelling may develop with disorders such as scleroderma and necrotizing vasculitis.

• *Arm swelling.* Unilateral or bilateral swelling of the arm aggravated by immobility and alleviated by elevation and exercise frequently results from trauma, such as a fracture, sprain, or strain. This swelling may also result from venous disorders, such as thrombophlebitis and superior vena cava syndrome, toxins such as those from insect bites, and treatments such as intravenous therapy.

• *Leg swelling.* Occurring unilaterally or bilaterally, swelling may affect just the foot, just the ankle, or the entire limb. Swelling may occur with conditions that disturb normal fluid balance or as a result of venous disorders, such as chronic venous insufficiency or thrombophlebitis; trauma, such as burns, fractures, sprains, or strains; certain bone disorders, such as osteomyelitis; and cardiac problems such as congestive heart failure.

Prolonged sitting, standing, or immobility may cause bilateral orthostatic swelling. This usually affects the foot, develops into pitting edema, and disappears with rest and elevation. Increased venous pressure during late pregnancy may cause a woman's ankles to swell.

Skin color changes. If your patient complains of a color change, such as pallor or erythema, explore his problem by asking appropriate questions from this list.

• When did he first notice the

change? Did the color change appear anywhere else first? Does it occur bilaterally?

• Is the color change constant or intermittent? If intermittent, what brings it on? Does anything make it better or worse?

• Does the affected area feel warm, cool, or the same as before the color changed? If he says warm or cool, ask if he feels any sensory changes, such as numbness, tingling, or throbbing. Ask him about any pain or itching that accompanies this change.

• Has this happened before? Has he recently had a fever, upper respiratory tract infection, joint pain, or rash?

Analyzing the chief complaint. Color changes in a limb include pallor and erythema. Pallor is usually associated with diminished blood flow, whereas erythema usually indicates acute inflammation, infection, or recent trauma. Neither are usually associated with degenerative joint disease.

• *Pallor.* This change usually develops in just one limb and may occur suddenly or gradually. It may result from decreased peripheral oxyhemoglobin—reflecting diminished peripheral blood flow associated with vasoconstriction, arterial occlusion, or low cardiac output. Transient peripheral vasoconstriction may occur with exposure to cold, causing nonpathologic pallor.

• *Erythema.* Dilated or congested blood vessels produce erythema—the most common chief complaint associated with skin inflammation and irritation. The color ranges from bright red in acute conditions to pale violet or brown in chronic conditions.

Erythema usually results from changes in the arteries, veins, and small vessels, which lead to increased small-vessel perfusion. Erythema also results from tissue damage or any change in supporting tissue that increases vessel visibility. For example, in an acute exacerbation of rheumatoid arthritis, erythema occurs over the affected joints, along with swelling, pain, and stiffness. In Raynaud's phenomenon, you'll find the skin on the hands and feet first blanches and cools after exposure to cold or stress, then becomes warm and purplish red. Thrombophlebitis is associated with erythema over the inflamed vein. Although erythema may occur over acutely inflamed joints, it may not be present with chronic inflammation.

Paresthesia. If the patient complains of sensory changes such as numbness or tingling, explore his problem by asking appropriate questions from this list.
• Ask when he first noticed the sensation. Did it begin gradually or suddenly? Where does it occur? Does it occur unilaterally? Is it constant or intermittent?
• Does anything make the paresthesia better or worse?
• Does he have any other loss of feeling, function, or movement? If so, where and to what degree?
• Has the area recently been injured?
• Is he taking any drugs? If so, what kind and how often?

Analyzing the chief complaint. Paresthesia — an abnormal sensation such as numbness, burning, pricking, or tingling felt along peripheral nerve pathways — usually isn't painful. It may develop suddenly or gradually and may be permanent or transient.
A common chief complaint of

many neurologic disorders, paresthesia also results from some systemic disorders, such as occlusive vascular diseases, hyperventilation syndrome, and vitamin B_6 deficiency, as well as from some drugs, such as chemotherapeutic agents.

In some cases, swelling can create pressure on a nerve, causing a loss of sensation in a distal area. Compression of nerves or blood vessels by a tumor or fracture can also cause a loss of feeling. The sensory changes reflect damage to or irritation of the parietal lobe, thalamus, spinothalamic tract, or spinal or peripheral nerves — the circuit responsible for transmitting and interpreting sensory stimuli.

Muscle spasm. If your patient complains of muscle spasm, explore his problem by asking appropriate questions from this list.
• When did he first experience the muscle spasm? Did it start gradually or suddenly? How often does it occur, and how long does it last? Is it constant or intermittent?
• Does anything make it better or worse?
• Ask if he has any accompanying symptoms, such as numbness, tingling, weakness, or pain.
• Ask him if he's taking any drugs. If so, what kind and how often?

Analyzing the chief complaint. Strong, painful muscular contractions, muscle spasm occurs most often in the calf and foot. Frequently precipitated by movement, muscle spasm can usually be relieved by slowly stretching the muscle.

Spasm typically results from simple muscle fatigue, exercise, or pregnancy. It may also occur in neuromuscular disorders such as spinal infections and amyotrophic lateral sclerosis as well as in electrolyte imbalances such as dehydration and hypocalcemia. If your patient has frequent or unrelieved spasm in many muscles, accompanied by paresthesia in his hands and feet, the problem may be hypocalcemic tetany. Certain drugs — diuretics and corticosteroids, for example — cause muscle spasm too.

Changes in mobility or function. If your patient complains of a change in limb mobility or function, explore his problem by asking appropriate questions from this list.
• When did he first notice the change? Is it unilateral or bilateral? Is the problem in the same area where he first noticed it?
• Did the change occur suddenly or gradually? Is it constant or intermittent? If intermittent, how often and when does it occur?
• Has he noticed any stiffness or muscle weakness? Does he feel pain? If so, ask him to describe it.
• What improves or worsens his condition?
• Ask if the change interferes with his normal routine. If it does, to what degree?
• Ask if he needs devices to assist or support him. If so, determine what kind and how often he uses them.
• Ask him if he's taking any drugs. If so, what kind and how often?

Analyzing the chief complaint. Mobility and function changes include joint stiffness, nontraumatic deformity, muscle weakness, muscle spasticity, and paralysis. They can result from pain, scar tissue, bony overgrowths, or other causes. Try to determine if your patient has an acute or chronic problem.
• *Joint stiffness.* Occurring with all arthropathies, morning joint stiffness is most commonly associated with rheumatoid arthritis. After

arising, the patient will be stiff for at least 30 minutes, with the stiffness easing as the day progresses. A joint also may become less mobile because of pain, muscle weakness, joint pathology, or prolonged patient immobility.
• *Nontraumatic deformity.* A slow-growing mass such as a tumor or gradual bony enlargement that occurs in a degenerative joint disease may cause limb deformity. With degenerative joint disease, the patient's limitation will depend on the joints involved and the progression of the disease. A patient with a flexion contracture of the hand, for instance, won't be able to extend his fingers.
• *Muscle weakness.* Caused by nerve degeneration or injury, or by altered chemical regulation at the neuromuscular junction or in the muscle itself, muscle weakness can affect a limb's ability to move or function. Such weakness occurs in neurologic and musculoskeletal disorders, metabolic conditions such as hypokalemia, endocrine disorders such as hypothyroidism, and cardiovascular disorders. Prolonged immobilization and prolonged use of certain drugs such as corticosteroids also can produce muscle weakness.
• *Muscle spasticity.* Excessive muscle tone with increased resistance to stretching and heightened reflexes, muscle spasticity results from an upper motor neuron lesion. It occurs most often in the arms and legs. Disorders commonly associated with muscle spasticity include cerebrovascular accident, multiple sclerosis, amyotrophic lateral sclerosis, and spinal cord injury. Long-term spasticity results in muscle fibrosis and contractures.
• *Paralysis.* A total loss of voluntary motor function, paralysis can be local or widespread, symmetrical or

asymmetrical, transient or permanent, and spastic or flaccid. You'll
usually find it classified according to
location and severity — such as para-
plegia, quadriplegia, or hemiplegia.

Paralysis results from severe cor-
tical or pyramidal tract damage and
is associated with cerebrovascular
disorders, degenerative neuromuscular disorders, trauma, tumors, and
central nervous system infection.
Acute paralysis may be an early indicator of a life-threatening disorder, such as Guillain-Barré
syndrome. In some patients, incom-
plete paralysis with profound weakness may precede total paralysis.

Physical assessment
When performing your physical assessment, keep in mind the basic
anatomy of the limbs and the normal assessment findings. (See *Arms
and legs: Normal findings.*)

You'll usually perform your inspection and palpation of the limbs
simultaneously. How much you use
these techniques and which limb
you examine will depend on your
patient's chief complaint. In some
cases, special function tests will follow your inspection and palpation.

As part of the examination, you'll
have the patient sit, stand, lie down,
and walk — unless his condition pro-
hibits this. As you examine the patient, compare both sides of his
body for symmetry and watch his
face closely for signs of discomfort
or pain.

Inspection. With the patient lying
down, sitting, or standing, quickly
inspect his affected limb for position, size, color, and shape. Look for
swelling, ecchymoses, abrasions, injuries, muscle atrophy, masses, and
breaks in skin integrity, such as ulcers. Punctures, ecchymoses, abrasions, or hematomas suggest

Arms and legs: Normal findings

Inspection
Normal findings include:
☐ no gross deformities
☐ symmetrical body parts
☐ good body alignment
☐ no involuntary movements
☐ a smooth gait
☐ active range of motion in all muscles and joints
☐ no pain with active range of motion
☐ no visible swelling or inflammation
of joints or muscles
☐ equal bilateral limb length and symmetrical muscle mass.

Palpation
Normal findings include:
☐ a normal shape with no swelling or
tenderness
☐ equal bilateral muscle tone, texture,
and strength
☐ no involuntary contractions or
twitching
☐ equally strong bilateral pulses.

damage to underlying structures
and should be assessed further.

With the patient standing, note
his build, posture, and bone structure. Observe him from the back,
sides, and front. Looking for bony
prominences, muscle mass, joint
structure, and symmetry, observe
the shoulder, elbow, wrist, hand,
and fingers of a patient with an arm
or hand complaint. Observe the hip,
knee, ankle, foot, and toes of a patient with a leg or foot complaint.
Are his knees in a direct line between his hips and ankles? Are both
feet flat on the floor, pointing directly in front of him?

If you suspect a discrepancy in
limb length, measure the limbs. To
do so, place the patient in the su-

Using reference points to measure limb circumference

To ensure accurate and consistent circumference measurements, measure with the limbs fully extended, use the same reference points each time, and measure the same distance from the reference points each time.

Use the olecranon process as your reference point on the arm and the patella as your reference point on the leg.

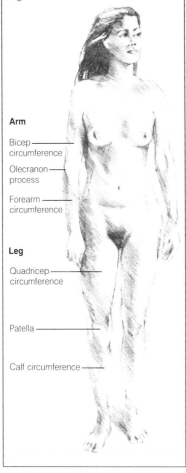

Arm

Bicep circumference

Olecranon process

Forearm circumference

Leg

Quadricep circumference

Patella

Calf circumference

pine position on a flat surface with his arms or legs fully extended and his shoulders or hips adducted. Measure each arm from the acromion process to the tip of the middle finger. If you're measuring the legs, start at the anterior superior iliac spine and measure to the medial malleolus, with the measuring tape crossing at the medial side of the knee. Note any disparity greater than 2½″ (1 cm) between sides.

If you detect swelling, asymmetry, or muscle rigidity, measure the circumference of the affected limb and compare it with that of the contralateral limb. To ensure that you measure corresponding locations on contralateral limbs, use reference points (see *Using reference points to measure limb circumference*). On each arm, measure an equal distance from the reference point to the area where you measure limb circumference. Follow the same procedure to measure the legs. Note any difference in measurements of corresponding areas.

While the patient walks, observe his gait, locomotion, coordination, and range of motion (ROM). Note any irregular, asymmetrical, or unsteady movements — including foot dragging or a limp (for a leg complaint) and decreased arm swing (for an arm complaint). Also note any signs of discomfort or pain.

Have the patient squeeze your hand or press his toes against your hand and wiggle his fingers or toes. Also have him attempt to perform full ROM exercises with the affected limb. If he's weak or unable to do this, help him with passive ROM exercises. (See *Assessing range of motion*.) Be careful not to force a joint into a painful position. Look for swelling and deformity; check the condition of the surrounding tissues.

(Text continues on page 167.)

Assessing range of motion

Shoulders
To assess forward flexion and backward extension, have the patient bring his straightened arm forward and up, and then behind him.

Forward flexion
180°

Backward extension
50° to 60°

Assess abduction and adduction by asking the patient to bring his straightened arm to the side and up, and then in front of him.

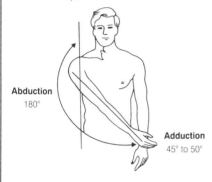

Abduction
180°

Adduction
45° to 50°

To assess external and internal rotation, have the patient abduct his arm with his elbow bent. Then ask him first to place his hand behind his head, then behind the small of his back.

External rotation
90°

Internal rotation
90°

Elbows
Assess flexion by having the patient bend his arm and attempt to touch his shoulder. Assess extension by having him straighten his arm.

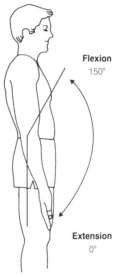

Flexion
150°

Extension
0°

To assess pronation and supination, hold the patient's elbow in a flexed position and ask him to rotate his arm until his palm faces the floor, then rotate his arm back until his palm faces upward.

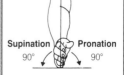

Supination
90°

Pronation
90°

(continued)

Assessing range of motion *(continued)*

Wrists

To assess flexion, ask the patient to bend his wrist downward; assess extension by having him straighten his wrist. To assess hyperextension, ask him to bend his wrist upward.

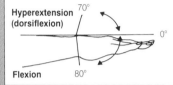

Assess radial and ulnar deviation by asking the patient to move his hand first toward the radial side, then toward the ulnar side.

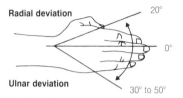

Fingers

To assess abduction and adduction, have the patient first spread his fingers and then bring them together. There should be 20 degrees between the fingers in abduction; in adduction, the fingers should touch.

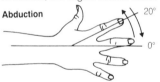

To assess extension and flexion, ask the patient first to straighten his fingers and then to make a fist with his thumb remaining straight.

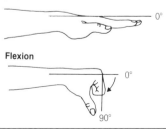

Thumbs

Assess extension by asking the patient to straighten his thumb. To assess flexion, ask him to bend his thumb, first at the top joint (the interphalangeal joint), then at the bottom joint (the metacarpophalangeal joint).

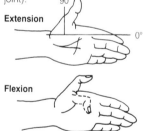

Assess adduction by having him extend his hand, bringing his thumb to the index finger, then the little finger.

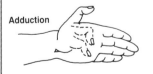

Hips

Assess flexion by asking the patient to bend his knee to his chest while keeping his back straight. If the patient has undergone total hip replacement, don't perform this movement without the surgeon's permission because the motion can cause the prosthesis to dislocate.

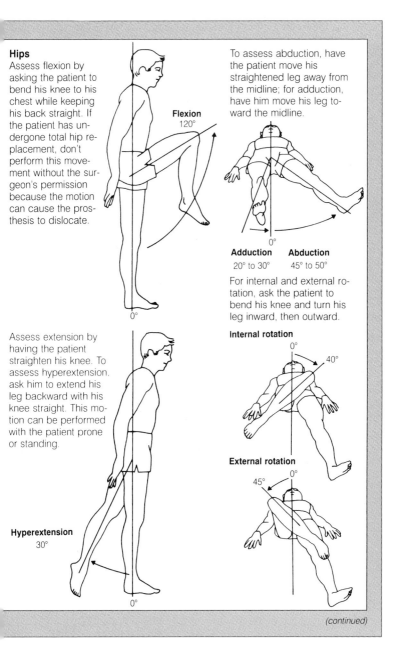

Flexion
120°

0°

Assess extension by having the patient straighten his knee. To assess hyperextension, ask him to extend his leg backward with his knee straight. This motion can be performed with the patient prone or standing.

Hyperextension
30°

0°

To assess abduction, have the patient move his straightened leg away from the midline; for adduction, have him move his leg toward the midline.

0°

Adduction   **Abduction**
20° to 30°   45° to 50°

For internal and external rotation, ask the patient to bend his knee and turn his leg inward, then outward.

Internal rotation
0°
40°

External rotation
45°   0°

(continued)

Assessing range of motion *(continued)*

Knees
Ask the patient to straighten his leg at the knee to demonstrate extension; ask him to bend his knee and bring his foot up to touch his buttock to demonstrate flexion.

Ankles and feet
Have the patient demonstrate plantar flexion by bending his foot downward, and hyperextension by bending his foot upward.

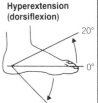

Hyperextension (dorsiflexion)   20°   0°

Plantar flexion   45° to 50°

To assess eversion and inversion, ask the patient to point his toes. Have him turn his foot inward, then outward.

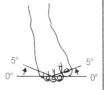

5°   5°
0°   0°

Eversion   **Inversion**

To assess forefoot adduction and abduction, stabilize the patient's heel while he turns his foot first inward, then outward.

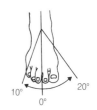

10°   20°
0°

Abduction   **Adduction**

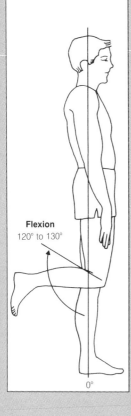

Flexion
120° to 130°

0°

Toes
Assess extension and flexion by asking the patient to straighten and then curl his toes. Then check hyperextension by asking him to straighten his toes and point them upward.

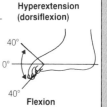

Hyperextension (dorsiflexion)
40°
0°
40°
Flexion

Note any signs of discomfort, pain, or stiffness.

Palpation. Use palpation to detect abnormalities, such as tenderness, crepitus, deformity, loss of bone integrity, and foreign or loose bodies under the skin.

Joints. Typically you'll palpate the joints of the affected limb during ROM exercises. Note any abnormal mobility; with or without crepitus, consider it a sign of a fracture. Check for fine crepitus over a joint by palpating with your palm and fingertips. Fine crepitus may indicate roughened articular surfaces, possibly from erosion, or fine granulation tissue, possibly caused by chronic inflammatory arthritis.

Muscles. Palpate muscles of the affected limb for tenderness. Also note tight cordlike muscles that may bulge slightly, indicating muscle spasm. If the patient has frequent or unrelieved muscle spasms and paresthesia, try to elicit Chvostek's and Trousseau's signs (see *Eliciting Chvostek's and Trousseau's signs*, page 168). If you note a dramatically different muscle shape or extreme bulging — especially after trauma — suspect a muscle rupture.

Skin. Using the back of your hand, check the temperature of the affected limb and compare it with the corresponding area on the other limb. Note excessively moist or dry skin.

Palpating the skin's texture may help you identify an abnormality. For example, tight shiny skin may cover an edematous joint, and smooth, shiny, hairless skin suggests an area of chronic poor circulation, as seen with chronic arterial insufficiency. Rough thickened skin, possibly with ulcerations, may indicate chronic venous insufficiency.

If you detect edema, check for pitting by pressing your fingertips over the swollen area for 30 seconds. (Make sure you're pressing over a bone.) Release your fingertips and measure the depth of the pitting. Also, mark the exact location to aid in later comparisons.

Assess capillary refill by momentarily pressing the nail beds of the toes or fingers. When you release the pressure, note the amount of time it takes for the color to return. Normal refill time is less than 3 seconds.

Pulses. To assess circulation in the affected limb, palpate your patient's peripheral pulses. Check the brachial and radial pulses for an arm or hand complaint and the femoral, popliteal, posterior tibial, and dorsalis pedis pulses for a leg or foot complaint. (See *Palpating peripheral pulses*, pages 170 and 171.)

Arms. For an arm or hand complaint, gently palpate the circumference of the arm from the shoulder to the fingers, using both hands. Then beginning at the shoulder, palpate the humerus. Next, starting at the top of the sternum, palpate along the clavicle to the shoulder joint. Be sure to check the acromioclavicular and sternoclavicular joints for continuity, pain, and malposition. Any stress to the arm may injure the clavicle and supporting structures.

If you suspect infection or inflammation in the patient's arm, palpate the axillae for enlarged lymph nodes. Using your nondominant hand to support the patient's arm, place your other hand as high as possible in the axilla. Gently press the soft tissue against the chest wall and muscles surrounding the axilla.

Eliciting Chvostek's and Trousseau's signs

When your patient complains of muscle spasms and paresthesia in his limbs, try eliciting Chvostek's and Trousseau's signs — indications of tetany associated with calcium deficiency. Follow the procedures described below, keeping in mind the discomfort they typically cause.

If you detect these signs, notify the doctor immediately. Watch the patient closely for laryngospasm, monitor his cardiac status, and if necessary prepare for resuscitation measures.

Chvostek's sign

Tap the patient's facial nerve just in front of the earlobe and below the zygomatic arch, or between the zygomatic arch and the corner of the mouth. A positive response, indicating latent tetany, ranges from simple mouth-corner twitching to twitching of all facial muscles on the side tested. Although simple twitching may be normal in some patients, a more pronounced response usually indicates a positive Chvostek's sign.

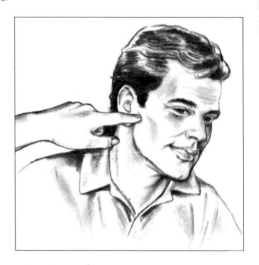

Trousseau's sign

Wrap a blood pressure cuff around the patient's arm, just above the antecubital area, and inflate it until you block the arm's blood supply. Watch the patient's hand for thumb adduction, followed by metacarpophalangeal flexion, interphalangeal joint extension (with the fingers together), finger adduction, and wrist and elbow flexion. If you see this sequence, you've elicited a carpopedal spasm, a positive Trousseau's sign.

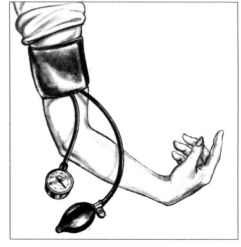

Also palpate his epitrochlear lymph nodes by placing your fingertips in the depression above the medial area of the elbow. Describe the lymph nodes according to their size, shape, consistency, mobility, and tenderness.

Legs. For a patient with a leg or foot complaint, you'll palpate much as you would for an arm or hand complaint. Start at the pelvis and work down toward the toes.

Inguinal lymph nodes are especially important to assess if the patient has redness and warmth in his legs, feet, or toes. Be sure to note the size, shape, consistency, mobility, and tenderness of the lymph nodes.

If you suspect a vascular problem, examine the legs for Homans' sign. Have the patient sit on the edge of the bed or lie on his back with his knee slightly flexed. Support his thigh with one hand and his foot with the other. Then firmly dorsiflex his ankle. A complaint of calf pain on dorsiflexion is a positive Homans' sign — possibly indicating deep vein thrombosis or thrombophlebitis.

Function tests. Based on your findings, you may need to continue assessing the affected limb by checking muscle strength, sensory response, and reflexes.

Muscle strength. Evaluate the patient's muscle strength by having him perform active ROM exercises against resistance (see *Testing muscle strength*, pages 172 and 173).

Sensory response. Assess your patient's sensory response to touch or pain. Starting at the bottom of the limb, gently stimulate the skin with the sharp end of a pin. Next, use your fingerpad or the blunt end of the pin to see if the patient can dis-

tinguish between sharp and dull sensations. Test his sense of touch by lightly brushing his skin with a piece of cotton or your fingertips. Each time, ask him where you're touching him. Once or twice, just pretend to touch him to see if he can tell the difference.

Reflexes. If you suspect a neurologic problem, assess the superficial reflexes in the affected limb. For a patient with a leg or foot complaint, test the cremasteric reflex in males and the plantar and Babinski's reflexes.

To elicit the cremasteric reflex, lightly stroke the inner aspect of the patient's upper thigh with a tongue depressor. The testis on the same side as the stimulus should rise. To test the plantar reflex, firmly stroke the lateral surface of the dorsal aspect of the foot with a firm, blunt object. The foot and toes should plantar flex. Babinski's reflex, the opposite of the plantar reflex, indicates pathology in adults.

Further assessment. As mentioned, you also may need to assess another part of the body. For example, to gather more information about pulses and peripheral circulation, you may need to quickly assess the heart and the carotid pulse. Or if your patient has motor or sensory problems, you may need to assess his head and neck for an injury. (See *Arms and legs: Interpreting your findings*, pages 174 and 175.)

Pediatric considerations
You'll have to modify your approach when your patient is a child. For instance, his developmental stage will determine how or whether you ask him history questions and how you assess his ability to move his limbs. Place an infant or small child on his parent's lap during your examina-

Palpating peripheral pulses

To palpate a peripheral pulse, apply pressure with your index and middle fingers to the site. Press gently to avoid obliterating the pulse—especially in the legs, where pressure is low because of the distance from the heart. Note the rate, rhythm, contour, and strength for each pulse. Be sure to compare pulses bilaterally.

The following illustrations and explanations show where to palpate each of the peripheral pulses.

Brachial pulse
Position your fingers medial to the bicep tendon.

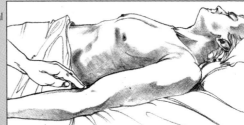

Radial pulse
Apply gentle pressure to the medial and ventral side of the wrist.

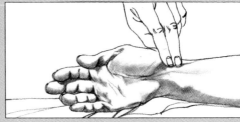

Femoral pulse
Press fairly hard at a point inferior to the inguinal ligament. For an obese patient, palpate the crease of the groin halfway between the pubic bone and the hip bone.

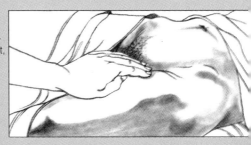

tion to ease the patient's anxiety.

Inspection. Because you won't be able to assess the gait of an infant, focus on his movements. How does he kick and wiggle his legs?

With a toddler under age 2, you'll normally find that his gait involves a wide support base. When assessing structure, remember that children ages 2 to 3½ commonly have knee deviations—knock-knee and

Popliteal pulse
Press firmly against the popliteal fossa.

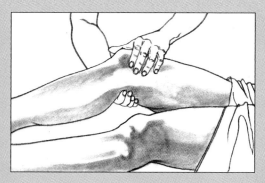

Posterior tibial pulse
Apply pressure behind and slightly below the medial malleolus of the ankle.

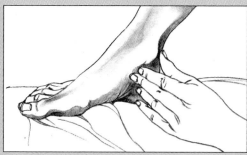

Dorsalis pedis pulse
Place your fingers on the medial dorsum of the foot while the patient points his toes. This pulse may prove difficult to palpate and so may appear to be absent in some healthy patients.

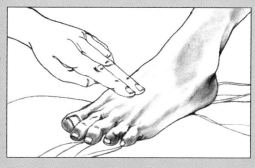

bowlegs, for instance. This may continue until a child turns 6.

Palpation. To ensure the patient's cooperation, always try to palpate the affected part of a limb last.

Function tests. If the patient can't follow directions, you can assess his muscle strength by observing his active and passive motions. For instance, watch him grasp objects and

(Text continues on page 176.)

Testing muscle strength

Assess your patient's motor function by testing his strength in the affected limb. Have him attempt normal range-of-motion movements against your resistance. If a muscle group seems weak, vary the amount of resistance to permit an accurate assessment. If necessary, position the patient so his limb doesn't have to resist gravity, and repeat the test.

ARM AND HAND MUSCLES

Deltoid
With the patient's arm fully extended, place one hand over his deltoid muscle and the other on his wrist. Have him abduct his arm to a horizontal position against your resistance; as he does, palpate for deltoid contraction.

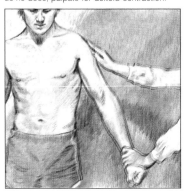

Biceps
With your hand on the patient's fist, have him flex his forearm against your resistance; observe for biceps contraction.

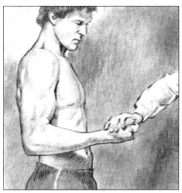

Triceps
Have the patient abduct and hold his arm midway between flexion and extension. Hold and support his arm at the wrist, and ask him to extend it against your resistance. Observe for triceps contraction.

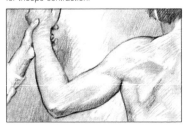

Dorsal interosseous
Have him extend and spread his fingers and resist your attempt to squeeze them together.

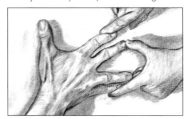

Forearm and hand (grip)
Have the patient grasp your middle and index fingers and squeeze them as hard as he can.

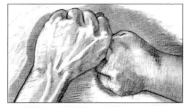

Rate muscle strength on a scale from 0 to 5:
0 = Total paralysis
1 = Visible or palpable contraction, but no movement
2 = Full muscle movement with force of gravity eliminated
3 = Full muscle movement against gravity, but no movement against resistance
4 = Full muscle movement against gravity; partial movement against resistance
5 = Full muscle movement against both gravity and resistance—normal strength

LEG AND FOOT MUSCLES

Psoas
While you support his leg, have the patient raise his knee and flex his hip against your resistance. Observe for psoas contraction.

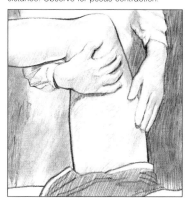

Quadriceps
Have the patient bend his knee slightly while you support his lower leg. Then ask him to extend his knee against your resistance; as he's doing so, palpate for quadriceps contraction.

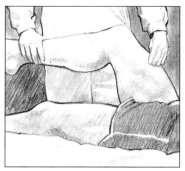

Gastrocnemius
With the patient on his side, support his foot and ask him to plantar-flex his ankle against your resistance. Palpate for gastrocnemius contraction.

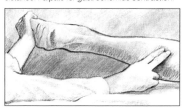

Anterior tibial
With the patient in the same position, place your hand on his foot and ask him to dorsiflex his ankle against your resistance.

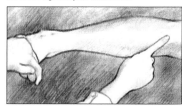

Extensor hallucis longus
With your finger on his great toe, have him dorsiflex the toe against your resistance. Palpate for extensor hallucis contraction.

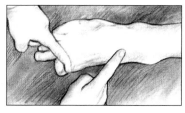

DIAGNOSTIC IMPRESSION

Arms and legs: Interpreting your findings

After you assess the patient, a group of findings may lead you to suspect a particular disorder. The chart below shows you some common groups of findings for the chief complaints of the arms and legs, along with the appropriate nursing diagnostic categories and probable causes.

CHIEF COMPLAINT AND FINDINGS	NURSING DIAGNOSTIC CATEGORIES	PROBABLE CAUSE
Pain		
• Throbbing pain • Crepitus • Decreased circulation • Decreased motion • Deformity • Ecchymosis • Paresthesia • Swelling	• Altered peripheral tissue perfusion • Impaired physical mobility • Impaired tissue integrity • Pain • Potential for infection	Fracture
• Shooting pain exacerbated by activity and relieved by rest; radiates down back of leg • Difficulty moving from sitting or standing position • Limping gait	• Activity intolerance • Pain • Potential for injury • Self-care deficit	Sciatica
Swelling		
• Bilateral swelling of legs • Chest tightness • Dyspnea • Hypotension • Inspiratory crackles • Nausea • Pallor • Palpitations • Pitting at the ankles • Tachypnea • Weight gain	• Activity intolerance • Altered tissue perfusion • Fluid volume excess • Impaired gas exchange	Congestive heart failure
• Bilateral swelling of legs; progresses slowly • Dilated neck veins • Edema in face and neck • Headache • Vertigo • Visual disturbances	• Altered tissue perfusion • Anxiety • Fluid volume excess • Potential for injury	Superior vena cava syndrome
Changes in color		
• Pallor with detectable line of demarcation separating cool, pale, cyanotic, and mottled skin from normal skin • Abrupt onset • Absent distal pulses	• Altered peripheral tissue perfusion • Pain • Potential for injury • Potential for trauma	Acute arterial occlusion

DIAGNOSTIC IMPRESSION

Arms and legs: Interpreting your findings (continued)

CHIEF COMPLAINT AND FINDINGS	NURSING DIAGNOSTIC CATEGORIES	PROBABLE CAUSE
Changes in color (continued)		
• Decreased capillary refill below line of demarcation • Intense intermittent claudication • Paresis, paresthesia • Severe pain		
• Erythema • Sudden onset • Exposure to irritant • Vesicles, blisters on exposed skin	• Anxiety • Body image disturbance • Impaired skin integrity • Knowledge deficit	Contact dermatitis
Paresthesia		
• Asymmetrical paresthesia, especially fingers and toes • Cramps, muscle weakness • Hyperactive deep tendon reflexes • Palpitations • Positive Chvostek's and Trousseau's signs • Twitching	• Potential for impaired gas exchange • Potential for injury • Tactile sensory-perceptual alterations	Hypocalcemic tetany
Muscle spasm		
• Ataxic gait • Contractures, dysarthria • Emotional lability • Exacerbations of diplopia, blurred vision, paresthesia • Hyperreflexia • Incoordination • Tremor • Urinary dysfunction	• Body image disturbance • Impaired physical mobility • Potential for injury • Potential impaired gas exchange • Reflex incontinence • Self-care deficit	Multiple sclerosis
Changes in mobility		
• Diminished reflexes accompanied by severe low back pain radiating unilaterally to buttock, hip, foot • Muscle weakness and atrophy • Sensory changes	• Impaired physical mobility • Pain • Potential for injury	Lumbo-sacral herniated disk
• Loss of vibratory sense • Mild to sharp burning pain • Muscle weakness progressing to flaccid paralysis and atrophy • Paresthesia	• Activity intolerance • Altered role performance • Fatigue • Impaired physical mobility • Potential for disuse syndrome • Potential for injury • Self-care deficit	Peripheral neuropathy

transfer them from hand to hand.

Because infants and toddlers can't express themselves well and have poor sensory localization, sensory testing may be difficult to perform.

Try to assess the palmar grasp reflex for an infant with an arm or hand problem. For an infant with a leg or foot problem, assess the plantar grasp, Babinski's, and stepping reflexes. Up to 18 months of age, a positive Babinski's reflex is normal.

Geriatric considerations

Although rapid assessment of an elderly patient is similar to that for any adult, the findings may differ. For example, his age may cause a blunted pain response. He may also display a slower reaction time and possibly irregular, somewhat uncoordinated movements because of decreased nerve conduction and muscle tone.

Remember that the elderly patient may tire more easily than other adults, so allow time for him to rest.

Inspection. An elderly patient may exhibit a loss of muscle mass and strength, as well as fine tremors. You may note an abnormal gait with an uneven rhythm and a wide support base. He also may take short steps because of a loss of muscle strength and coordination, a fear of falling, arthritic pain, peripheral neuropathy, or poor vision. Plus, his gait may be affected by medications.

Observe for any mild unilateral weakness, such as a clumsy hand or dragging foot, which could result from a small cerebrovascular accident. A shuffling, accelerating gait,

"pill rolling" hand tremors, and cogwheel rigidity of the extremities may accompany Parkinson's disease. Arthritis may produce a partially adducted and flexed hip joint, as well as limited ROM during rotation and hyperextension.

Palpation. When assessing an elderly patient's pulse, you may note swollen limbs or a change in the character of the pulses, possibly caused by peripheral vascular disease or cardiovascular disease. You may also note diminished peripheral pulses from a decrease in peripheral circulation.

Suggested readings

Cardona, V., et al. *Trauma Nursing: From Resuscitation Through Rehabilitation.* Philadelphia: W.B. Saunders Co., 1988.

Howell, E., et al. *Comprehensive Trauma Nursing.* Glenville, Ill.: Scott, Foresman and Co., 1988.

Karren, K.J., and Hafen, B.Q. *First Responder: A Skills Approach,* 3rd ed. Englewood, Colo.: Morton Publishing Co., 1990.

Kenner, C.V., et al. *Critical Care Nursing.* Boston: Little, Brown & Co., 1990.

Malasanos, L., et al. *Health Assessment,* 4th ed. St. Louis: C.V. Mosby Co., 1989.

Morton, P. *Health Assessment in Nursing.* Springhouse, Pa.: Springhouse Corp., 1989.

Potter, P. *Pocket Nurse Guide to Physical Assessment,* 2nd ed. St. Louis: C.V. Mosby Co., 1990.

Trauma Nursing Core Course Manual (TNCC). Emergency Nurses Association. Award Printing Co., Chicago, Ill. 1987.

SELF-TEST

Test your rapid assessment knowledge and skills at your own pace by answering the multiple-choice questions on pages 178 to 180. Answers appear on page 180.

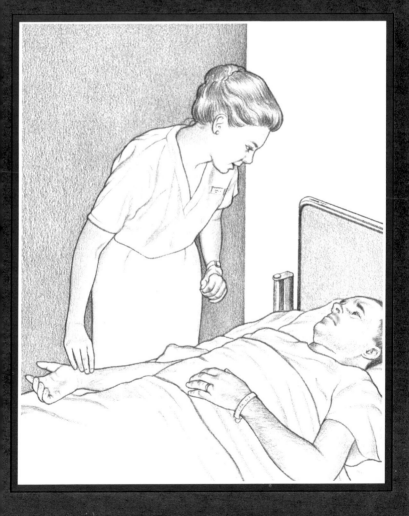

1. *When using the abdominal thrust technique on a conscious patient, you should:*
a. place him in the supine position and kneel astride his thighs to deliver the thrusts.
b. have him stand or sit up and wrap your arms around his waist to deliver the thrusts.
c. sit him up and deliver four forceful blows between his shoulder blades, then wrap your arms around his waist to deliver the thrusts.
d. try to ventilate him after you've administered six to ten thrusts.

2. *Margaret Fenton, a 37-year-old patient admitted to the hospital for tests to rule out lung cancer, is having trouble swallowing. On tracheal palpation, you discover a narrow space on the left side between the trachea and the sternocleidomastoid muscle. This may indicate:*
a. poor posture.
b. a congenital malformation.
c. a normal trachea.
d. a pulmonary or mediastinal mass.

3. *When you enter 67-year-old Stacy Wilson's room, she complains that she's spitting up blood when she coughs. You take a quick health history that includes:*
a. the history of the present problem, medications, review of systems, and recent major operations.
b. the history of the present problem, allergies, medications, and recent major operations.
c. the history of the present problem, medications, family history, psychosocial history, and review of systems.
d. the history of the present problem, allergies, medications, review of systems, and recent major operations.

4. *When questioning Mrs. Wilson about medications, you should ask if she has been taking:*
a. pills or liquid medicine.
b. anticoagulants.
c. antacids.
d. antibiotics.

5. *Why shouldn't you palpate both carotid arteries at the same time?*
a. You can't assess the pulse accurately unless you palpate the arteries one at a time.
b. You may cause transient hypertension.
c. You may cause severe bradycardia.
d. You may cause severe tachycardia.

6. *Why should an infant be quiet and seated upright when you assess his fontanels?*
a. The mother will have less trouble holding a quiet, upright infant.
b. Lying down can cause the fontanels to recede, making assessment more difficult.
c. The infant can breathe more easily when sitting up.
d. Lying down and crying can cause the fontanels to bulge.

7. *The pneumonic device PQRST stands for:*
a. practices, quantity, region, source, and tone.
b. provoking or palliative factors, quality or quantity, region or radiation, severity, and timing.
c. provoking factor, quality or quantity, region or radiation, source, and tone.
d. practices, quantity, region, severity, and time.

8. *At shift report, you learn that Carl Stenton, a 47-year-old recovering from abdominal surgery, is agitated and has been complaining. The nurse giving the report thinks he needs his pain medication. Before getting it, you go to his room and note that he's agitated, flushed, sweating, and short of breath. Should you give him his pain medication?*
a. yes
b. no

9. *What's the reason for your answer to the previous question?*
a. Mr. Stenton may have a pulmonary embolism.
b. Mr. Stenton is a chronic complainer.
c. Mr. Stenton is in pain.
d. Mr. Stenton probably has flatus.

10. *The ear canal of an infant or young child:*
a. slants upward.
b. slants downward.
c. is horizontal.
d. slants backward.

11. *When performing a rapid assessment of a young child, you should inspect, then:*
a. percuss.
b. palpate.
c. auscultate.

12. *What's the reason for your answer to the previous question?*
a. Your touch may calm the child.
b. The child may cry as the assessment proceeds, making auscultation difficult.
c. Your touch may frighten the child.
d. Your hands or the stethoscope may feel cold, making the child recoil.

13. *When you enter the room of 28-year-old Brent Eastman, a patient with cystic fibrosis, you find him short of breath. Your first step should be to:*
a. elevate the head of his bed.
b. take vital signs.
c. obtain a brief health history.
d. call for help.

14. *Which of the following is true of crackles?*
a. They're grating sounds.
b. They're high-pitched, musical squeaks.
c. They're low-pitched noises that sound like snoring.
d. They may be fine, medium, or coarse.

15. *Gurgles indicate:*
a. constricted airways.
b. fluid in the larger upper airways.
c. thick secretions partially obstructing the upper airways.
d. fluid in the alveoli.

16. *On assessment, you find that Mr. Eastman has Grade 3 dyspnea, which is defined as shortness of breath resulting from:*
a. walking a short distance.
b. performing normal activities of daily living.
c. sitting up.
d. lying down.

17. *When placing your hands to perform chest compressions on an adult, which landmark should you use?*
a. the nipple line
b. the sternal notch
c. the xiphoid process
d. the supraclavicular line

18. *What's the ratio of chest compressions to ventilations when one rescuer performs cardiopulmonary resuscitation (CPR) on an adult?*
a. 15:1
b. 15:2
c. 12:1
d. 12:2

19. *What's the ratio of chest compressions to ventilations when performing CPR on a child?*
a. 5:1
b. 5:2
c. 15:1
d. 15:2

20. *The most common source of airway obstruction is:*
a. a foreign object.
b. saliva or mucus.
c. the tongue.
d. edema.

21. *Don't stop CPR until:*
a. the patient shows signs of returning consciousness.
b. the patient fails to respond after 8 minutes of CPR.
c. you feel tired.
d. you can turn CPR over to someone else.

22. *When performing an assessment of a patient suspected of having cardiac disease, palpate the pulse for:*
a. 15 seconds.
b. 30 seconds.
c. 60 seconds.
d. 120 seconds.

23. *Which pulse should you palpate during a rapid assessment?*
a. radial
b. brachial
c. femoral
d. carotid

24. *Tachycardia can result from:*
a. vagal stimulation.
b. vomiting, anger, or suctioning.
c. fear, pain, or anger.
d. stress, pain, or vomiting.

25. *To avoid recording an erroneously low systolic blood pressure because of a failure to recognize an ausculatory gap, you should:*
a. have the patient lie down while you take his blood pressure.
b. inflate the cuff to at least 200 mm Hg.
c. take blood pressure readings in both arms.
d. inflate the cuff at least another 20 mm Hg after the radial pulse becomes unpalpable.

26. *Cardiac pain can radiate to all of the following* except *the:*
a. abdomen.
b. shoulder.
c. jaw and neck.
d. arm and wrist.

27. *You can auscultate heart sounds more easily if your patient is:*
a. supine.
b. on his right side.
c. holding his breath.
d. leaning forward.

28. *Which statement regarding heart sounds is correct?*
a. S_1 and S_2 sound equally loud over the entire cardiac area.
b. S_1 and S_2 sound fainter at the apex.
c. S_1 and S_2 sound fainter at the base.
d. S_1 is loudest at the apex; S_2 is loudest at the base.

29. *Which sequence should you follow when assessing the abdomen?*
a. inspection, percussion, auscultation, palpation
b. auscultation, inspection, percussion, palpation
c. inspection, auscultation, percussion, palpation
d. auscultation, inspection, palpation, percussion ·

30. *When examining a patient with abdominal pain, assess:*
a. any quadrant first.
b. the symptomatic quadrant first.
c. the symptomatic quadrant last.
d. the symptomatic quadrant either second or third.

31. *Hyperactive bowel sounds can result from all of the following* except:
a. hunger.
b. paralytic ileus.
c. intestinal obstruction.
d. diarrhea.

32. *When should you check a patient with abdominal pain for rebound tenderness?*
a. near the beginning of the examination
b. before doing anything else
c. anytime during the examination
d. at the end of the examination

ANSWERS

1. b	**6.** d	**11.** c	**16.** b	**21.** d	**26.** a	**31.** b
2. d	**7.** b	**12.** b	**17.** c	**22.** c	**27.** d	**32.** d
3. b	**8.** b	**13.** a	**18.** b	**23.** d	**28.** d	
4. b	**9.** a	**14.** d	**19.** a	**24.** c	**29.** c	
5. c	**10.** a	**15.** c	**20.** c	**25.** d	**30.** c	

INDEX

182

INDEX

i refers to an illustration; t refers to a table.

i refers to an illustration; *t* refers to a table.

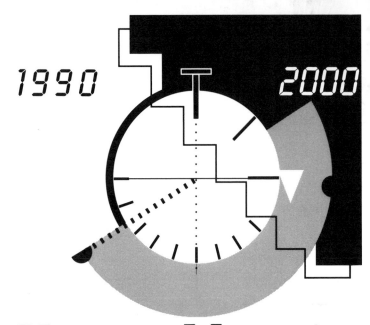

1990   2000

Nursing Magazine
In the future as in the past...

You can rely on *Nursing* magazine to keep your skills sharp and your practice current—with award—winning nursing journalism.

Each monthly issue is packed with expert advice on the legal, ethical, and personal issues in nursing, plus up-to-the-minute...

- Drug information—warnings, new uses, and approvals

- Assessment tips

- Emergency and acute care advice

- New treatments, equipment, and dis findings

- Photostories and skill sharpeners

- AIDS updates

- Career tracks and trends

SAVE 38%
Enter your subscription today.
